LASERS

INVENTION TO
APPLICATION

JOHN R. WHINNERY
Symposium Chairman

JESSE H. AUSUBEL
H. DALE LANGFORD
Editors

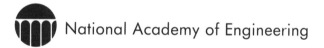

National Academy of Engineering

NATIONAL ACADEMY PRESS
WASHINGTON, D.C., 1987

NATIONAL ACADEMY PRESS
2101 Constitution Avenue, NW
Washington, DC 20418

NOTICE: The National Academy of Engineering was established in 1964, under the charter of the National Academy of Sciences, as a parallel organization of outstanding engineers. It is autonomous in its administration and in the selection of its members, sharing with the National Academy of Sciences the responsibility for advising the federal government. The National Academy of Engineering also sponsors engineering programs aimed at meeting national needs, encourages education and research, and recognizes the superior achievements of engineers. Dr. Robert M. White is president of the National Academy of Engineering.

Funds for the National Academy of Engineering's symposium "Twenty-Five Years of the Laser" were provided by the Academy's Technological Leadership Program.

Library of Congress Catalog Card Number 87-042941

ISBN 0-309-03776-X

Printed in the United States of America

First Printing, September 1987
Second Printing, April 1988

Preface and Acknowledgments

Month by month the practical applications of lasers are more evident. They provide the music in our homes and print the documents in our offices. They are integral to our systems for telecommunications and national security and, increasingly, medical care. As this report vividly portrays, the laser story is one of harmony between engineering and science, industry and universities, the impulse of the inventor and the needs of society. It is a story we should understand as we seek to provide fertile ground for discovery and to reap greater benefits from research.

Anthony Siegman and John Whinnery urged the National Academy of Engineering (NAE) to take note in 1985 of the 25th anniversary of the invention of the laser. With their assistance, we organized a symposium commemorating discoveries that brought this technological star into our midst and exploring where laser light might lead us in the future. The symposium was so successful that we decided to seek to capture the essence of the presentations in a publication that might bring the excitement and intensity of the laser story to a broader audience. This report is the result.

We are grateful to the authors for translating what were often highly visual presentations into words and images that can be conveyed in printed form. John Whinnery guided the endeavor with imagination and affection. NAE staff members Jesse Ausubel and Dale Langford provided effective support and editorial assistance.

I hope the readers of this report will gain a greater appreciation of one of the seminal inventions of our era and the many dimensions of our research and industrial institutions that can contribute to technological leadership. Let us emulate the invention and application of the laser many times over in harnessing technology to increase fundamental knowledge and promote economic growth.

ROBERT M. WHITE, *President*
National Academy of Engineering

Contents

LASERS

INVENTION TO
APPLICATION

The Laser: Still Young at 25?

Anthony E. Siegman

The first laser device was operated just over 25 years ago. In the subsequent two-and-a-half decades, laser devices of many diverse types have produced an enviable record of accomplishments in fundamental science, applied technology, medicine, and even home entertainment. Although not yet of the economic importance of conventional electronics, the laser industry is significant and growing.

This paper will provide a brief review of the history of the laser; describe some of the characteristics and performance capabilities of different types of laser devices; give a short introduction to the breadth and diversity of laser applications; and finally, summarize some of the exciting current accomplishments and possible future advances in laser technology.

LOOKING BACK 25 YEARS

To begin with the very early history or, perhaps, the mythology of the laser, the following passage from H. G. Wells's famous 1896 novel *The War of the Worlds,* about an invasion of Earth by Martians, gives a reasonably accurate description of how one might make and then use a laser.

In some way they [the Martians] are able to generate an intense heat in a chamber of practically absolute nonconductivity. . . . This intense heat they project in a parallel beam against any object they choose, by means of a polished parabolic mirror of unknown composition. . . .

The second part of this quotation then says:

However it is done, it is certain that a beam of heat is the essence of the matter. What is combustible flashes into flame at its touch, lead runs like water, it softens iron, cracks and melts glass, and when it falls upon water, that explodes into steam. . . .

To anyone who has seen the materials processing effects produced by even a medium-power laser beam, Wells's description, written at the turn of the century, will seem a remarkably accurate account of the effects of the beam from a modern carbon dioxide (CO_2) laser of perhaps a few kilowatts of power output. It should also come as no surprise that we now know, from our own space probes, that the natural atmosphere of the planet Mars consists primarily of carbon dioxide, and that, in fact, natural laser action, pumped by sunlight, occurs in the Martian atmosphere.

We of course do not really believe that Martian invaders brought CO_2 lasers with them to Earth a century ago, but the basic principles of stimulated emission from atoms or molecules were first recognized by Einstein, Ladenburg, and others in the 1930s. The first man-made device to use these principles came only in 1955, when Charles H. Townes of Columbia University operated the first ammonia beam *maser*—the acronym coined by Townes to stand for *m*icrowave *a*mplification by *s*timulated *e*mission of *r*adiation. This was closely followed by similar developments by N. G. Basov and A. M. Prokhorov in the Soviet Union. Townes's first maser was, of course, not an optical device, but a weak microwave oscillator at 24 GHz.

In the years that followed, many researchers gave much thought to the possibility of optical masers, or lasers. This process of development was much assisted by the concept of the continuously pumped three-level microwave maser developed by N. Bloembergen at Harvard University in 1956. In 1958 Townes and Arthur L. Schawlow of Bell Laboratories published a paper and patent application that gave a theoretical recipe for laser action. The first successful optical-frequency laser device, the pulsed ruby laser, was actually developed in 1960 by an industrial researcher, Theodore H. Maiman, in the Hughes Research Laboratories in Malibu, California.

Maiman produced this first laser action by placing silver mirrors directly on the end of a synthetic crystal of ruby, and then pumping or exciting this crystal with an intense flash of light from a standard photographic flash lamp. Maiman's pioneering advance was rapidly followed by the development of a number of other laser devices by the IBM and Bell Telephone Laboratories; in particular, the first continuously running, electrically pumped gas lasers were developed in the same year at

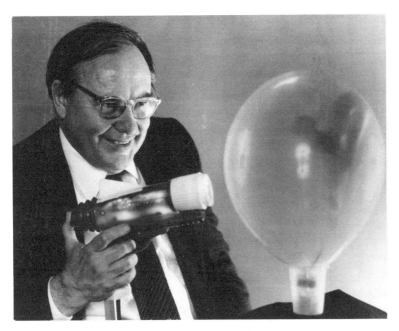

FIGURE 1   Arthur L. Schawlow demonstrating that a flash of red light from a small ruby laser breaks the dark-colored inner balloon without damaging the transparent outer balloon. This procedure exactly mimics the way laser light can be used to repair a detached retina inside the eyeball, make a weld inside a closed vacuum chamber, or trigger a chemical reaction inside a closed chemical cell. Photograph by Frans P. Alkemade.

Bell Labs. The laser field has been characterized ever since by the continual emergence of new and ever-surprising laser systems, a process that is still going on today.

Schawlow, one of the most distinguished scientists in the laser field, was a corecipient of the 1981 Nobel Prize for his work on laser spectroscopy. He was also the pioneer of the first edible laser: a glass cell full of unflavored gelatine, which he first operated as a laser and then ate. Figure 1 shows another of Schawlow's distinctive demonstrations.

HOW LASERS WORK

The construction of a laser begins with a collection of atoms. These atoms or molecules can be gaseous, liquid, or solid in form, but they are characterized, as are all atoms, by a set of discrete and distinctive quantum energy levels.

Next, some form of pumping process must be applied to these atoms. This pumping process can be accomplished in a great many ways. In all cases, however, its essential function is to excite or lift some of the laser atoms out of their lowest quantum energy level and into upper energy levels (see Figure 2).

If atoms can be excited into upper energy levels and, more importantly, a condition of population inversion can be achieved, in which more atoms are excited into some upper atomic level than into some lower atomic level, then laser action can occur. If a beam of light tuned to the transition frequency between those two levels is sent through the collection of atoms, that light beam will be amplified through the process of stimulated emission. Stimulated emission means simply that the electromagnetic fields in the light beam cause the atoms to drop down from the more heavily populated upper level into the less heavily populated lower level, giving up their energy to the light beam in the process, in phase (i.e., coherent) with the exciting field.

Next, a carefully aligned laser mirror is added at each end of the collection of atoms to form an optical resonator, in which the lightwave can bounce back and forth many times. If the round-trip gain in this resonator exceeds the round-trip losses due to absorption and finite mirror reflectivity, then the light signal in this laser cavity can build up to a coherent optical oscillation, exactly the same as in an audio frequency oscillator or a radio frequency transmitter.

The optical signal in this laser cavity can be highly monochromatic, or of a single frequency, or temporally coherent because it is a true coherent oscillator. It can also be highly directional (collimated) or spatially coherent because of the directional control produced by the two mirrors.

THE PRESENT STATUS OF LASERS

An enormous number of widely different types of laser devices have now been discovered (Table 1). They cover the wavelength range from shorter than 1,000 Å in the vacuum ultraviolet to longer than 800 μm in the far infrared or millimeter wavelength range. The list of laser materials covers essentially every form of matter, from simple gases and solids to liquids, plastics, flames, jet engine exhausts, and interplanetary space. Indeed, Schawlow's law, yet to be disproved experimentally, says that anything will lase (i.e., generate a beam of laser light) if it is hit hard enough. Of course, if something does not lase, then it was not hit hard enough.

The list of atoms in which laser action has been obtained

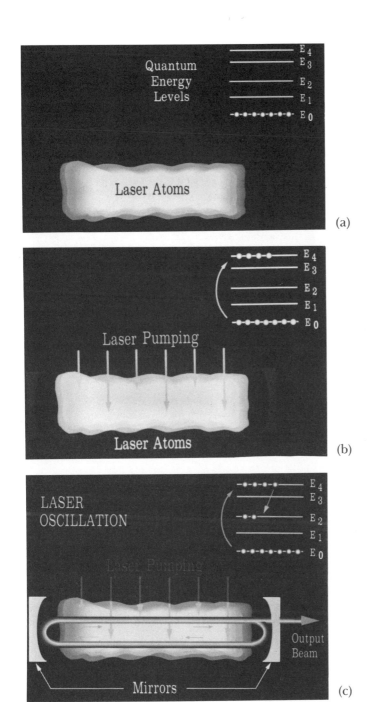

FIGURE 2 (a) A collection of laser atoms and their quantum energy levels. (b) The laser pumping process. (c) Stimulated emission and laser oscillation.

TABLE 1 Present Status of Lasers

Laser Characteristic	Present Status
Wavelength range	From longer than 800 μm to shorter than 150 Å
Laser materials	Gases: atoms, ions, molecules, excimers
	Liquids: organic dyes, H_2O solutions, Scotch whisky
	Solids: crystals, glasses, plastics, semiconductors, plasmas, flames, jet engine exhausts, interstellar space, planetary atmospheres
Laser atoms	More than 100 individual atoms and ions, innumerable molecular species
Laser transitions	More than 10^6 discrete laser lines
Peak powers	Greater than 10^{13} W
Average powers	Greater than 1 MW
Frequency stability	Few parts in 10^{14}
Pulsewidths	Less than 8 fs (8×10^{-15} s)
Tuning ranges	Greater than 200 Å (about 24,000 GHz)

covers essentially the entire periodic table, in both atomic and ionized forms, in addition to a virtually unlimited list of molecular species. The number of individual laser transitions is practically uncountable—there are, for example, more than 200 individually identifiable laser transitions between different quantum energy level pairs in the neutral neon atom alone. Therefore, the number of possible laser transitions is almost surely in the millions.

AN ELECTRONIC OLYMPIC GAMES?

One way of dramatizing the extraordinary capabilities of lasers might be through a sort of "Electronic Olympic Games," a set of competitive events to see which electronic devices—transistors, integrated circuits, vacuum tubes, or lasers—set the current performance records in generating the highest powers, the shortest pulses, the greatest frequency stability, the lowest noise figure, and other limits. How many gold medals might the laser, in particular, win in such a competition?

FREQUENCY RANGE, TUNING RANGE, AND BANDWIDTH

Laser devices of many different kinds will clearly win all the available gold, silver, and bronze medals for frequency range, tuning range, and instantaneous bandwidth. The frequency or wavelength range over which different kinds of lasers and masers can operate extends from the subaudio to the x-ray regions.

The fractional tuning range of most individual lasers is relatively small, limited by the atomic linewidth of the laser transition used. In absolute terms, however, the bandwidths or tuning ranges of many lasers still extend over tens to hundreds of gigahertz. So-called organic dye lasers, along with semiconductor lasers, can, in fact, be continuously tuned over linewidths of hundreds of angstroms; commercially available dye lasers with multiple dyes can be tuned continuously over essentially the entire visible and near-infrared spectral range. The applications of such lasers in chemistry and chemical diagnostics can be easily imagined.

Without going into further detail here, it should also be noted that an ordinary dye laser with a 200-Å spectral width has a frequency bandwidth sufficient to transmit the equivalent of one simultaneous telephone channel for every person on earth.

PEAK POWER

For setting peak power output records, laser devices also stand absolutely supreme, in large part because of their ability to generate very short pulses. Indeed, rather modest mode-locked lasers of tabletop size can easily produce optical pulses with instantaneous peak optical powers in excess of 10^{13} W, or several times the total installed electrical generating capacity of the United States—though these pulses last for only a few trillionths of a second.

These same laser pulses can then be focused into spots only a few optical wavelengths in diameter to produce peak power intensities of billions of watts per square centimeter—sufficient to tear atoms apart, break molecular bonds, produce intense nonlinear optical effects, and melt and vaporize any material. Even a small pulsed solid-state laser, for example, can readily drill or cut through steel, ceramic, diamond, or any other material.

CONTINUOUS POWER OUTPUT

The continuous or average powers available from certain laser devices are also impressive, although it is uncertain whether they exceed those available from all other high-power electronic devices, including klystrons, high-power triodes, and even motor generator sets. Of particular interest here, however, is the enormous diversity of pumping or excitation methods that can be used for producing laser action (Table 2). These include not merely electrical discharges of all kinds and optical pumping methods using almost any conceivable light source but also laser action in flames, plasmas, chemical reactions, focused sunlight, nuclear reactions, and nuclear explosions. Especially striking is the fact that several types of natural laser and maser action also occur (without mirrors) both in interstellar space and in planetary and solar atmospheres.

Particularly impressive in the context of high-power lasers are the chemical and gas-dynamic laser systems, which can convert the energy of a chemical reaction, or pure heat energy in gases, directly into coherent laser radiation with extremely high energy output. Figure 3 shows, for example, a large gas-dynamic laser built in the early 1970s. This laser burned a chemical fuel (cyanogen) in the lower chamber, and then sent the hot gases upward through supersonic expansion nozzles into the laser region to produce some hundreds of kilowatts or more of laser power. The water-cooled mirrors and mirror mounts are in the boxes at the end, and the hot gases are exhausted through the deflectors at the top. This is one of the few lasers that must be bolted down because it has thrust.

The rule of thumb for such chemical lasers is that the combustion of 1 kg of fuel can typically produce a sufficient number of excited molecules to provide several hundred kilojoules of coherent (though multiwavelength) laser output energy. A fuel supply of a few kilograms per second suffices, therefore, to power a 1-MW laser oscillator. Israeli scientists have

TABLE 2 Laser Pumping Methods

Pumping Method	Laser Action
Optical pumping	Laser materials pumped by flash lamps, arc lamps, tungsten lamps, exploding wires, light-emitting diodes, flames, focused sunlight, other lasers
Gas discharges	Direct electron and collisional excitation in glow discharges, arc discharges, hollow cathode discharges
Chemical reactions	Laser action following chemical mixing, flash photolysis, flame photolysis
Direct electrical	Direct electrical excitation in semiconductor injection lasers, electron beam-pumped solids and gases
Gas-dynamic lasers	Laser action derived from hot gases, supersonic expansions, shock fronts
Plasmas	Laser action in plasma pinches, laser-induced plasmas
Nuclear reactions	Fission fragment pumping of gas lasers
Nuclear explosions	Atomic bomb-pumped x-ray lasers
Natural lasers	Sunlight, interstellar radiation, particle beams

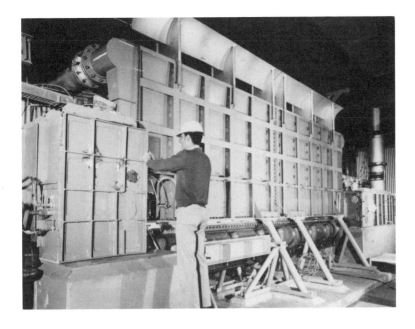

FIGURE 3   A large high-power gas-dynamic laser.

even developed a gasoline-fueled gas-dynamic laser, with the initial fuel mixture being ignited by an automobile spark plug.

EFFICIENCY

To be conservative, the laser should probably receive only a silver medal in the category of average power. Many commonly used lasers are also, unfortunately, far less efficient in the use of electrical input energy than would be desirable. The common small helium-neon laser has a typical operating efficiency of only a small fraction of a percent, although there are also useful types of gas and semiconductor lasers that have efficiencies of 60–70 percent from direct electrical input. In this category the laser would receive a bronze medal.

PULSEWIDTH

In the competition for generating the shortest possible pulses, however, the laser is second to none. The units for expressing the duration of a pulse scale downward in jumps of 1,000 from seconds to milliseconds, microseconds, nanoseconds, picoseconds—with 1 ps already shorter than any form of electronics can go—and finally down to femtoseconds, or units of 10^{-15} s.

One of the most astonishing recent accomplishments in laser technology has been the generation of fully coherent optical pulses as short as 8–10 fs. These have provided truly extraordinary new scientific capabilities for exciting, probing, and measuring internal processes in atoms and molecules, chemical reactions, biological processes, and solid-state physics—far beyond the time resolution that can be achieved electronically, now or in the near future.

FREQUENCY STABILITY AND SPECTRAL PURITY

Lasers may also be judged with respect to absolute frequency stability and spectral purity. For many decades the international standard for measurements of length has been not the historic meter bar but a visible wavelength derived from an incoherent, or nonlaser, gas-discharge light source. The international standard of time has been a microwave atomic clock, which is not quite but is almost a maser.

Certain laser oscillators can, however, have a spectral purity and absolute frequency stability so extraordinary that just in the past few years the international standards for both frequency and time have been, by definition, unified into a single laser device. That is, the new standards for both distance and time are now provided by a certain ultrastable laser oscillator transition located in the middle infrared region of the spectrum.

It is more than a little disconcerting to realize what this means: The goal of Albert A. Michelson and so many other distinguished physicists in the past—to make ever more precise measurements of the velocity of light—will no longer even be meaningful. Now that the basic standards of time and length are one and the same laser transition, the velocity of light, c, is reduced to a mere defined quantity: the numerical relationship between one wavelength and one period of this laser frequency. One can never again measure c.

ANTENNA BEAMWIDTH

The antenna properties or the antenna beamwidth of a laser beam are also important. The beam traveling back and forth inside a laser cavity is extraordinarily parallel or well collimated, and the beam outside the laser retains these extremely directional properties, spreading only slightly as it propagates (see Plate 1).

Such a laser beam thus provides a kind of "weightless string" that neither sags nor blows in the wind and so is extremely useful as an alignment tool for building construction, tunneling, pipe laying, and many other civil engineering works. This is, in fact, one of the simplest but most significant commercial applications for the laser, and the fortunes of some laser companies in the past have risen and fallen with the construction market.

In technical terms, the beam angle in radians for a collimated electromagnetic wave coming from an antenna is more or less equal to the number of wavelengths across the antenna aperture. For a visible laser beam and a diffraction-limited, 10-cm-diameter aperture—which is not at all difficult to achieve in practice—this means a beamwidth of 10 microradians; this means, in turn, that a laser easily has the ability to illuminate a spot not much more than a mile wide on the face of the moon. A microwave antenna with the same beamwidth would have to be several kilometers in diameter.

At present, laser antennas up to a meter in diameter are commonplace, for example, in satellite and lunar ranging systems. Given the narrow beams and high peak powers of lasers, laser radar echoes are routinely obtained from optical reflectors located on the moon, with accumulated range accuracies of a few centimeters in the distance to the moon. By making such laser-ranging measurements to a cooperative orbiting satellite simultaneously from multiple stations, it is possible first to determine the satellite orbit and its perturbations with great accuracy and then to determine the relative positions of the laser stations on earth, and thus to map the earth with comparable accuracy even across seas and oceans.

COMPUTING CAPABILITY

Laser light certainly will be—already is—of enormous importance in fiber-optic communications generally, including fiber-optic computer networks and communications between and within computers. Less well established, however, are the pure computing capabilities of lasers—the so-called photonic logic possibilities that may come in the future.

For sheer power in general computing, all the gold medals will probably continue to go to the silicon chip and its derivatives. The silver medals may well go to gallium arsenide or other new forms of ultrafast electronics rather than to any kind of "photonic computers."

Lasers can offer unique capabilities in certain specialized techniques that are more or less computational in nature, such as holography and certain kinds of image processing. However, the laser would receive at most a bronze medal in this area.

Out of a dozen or so major Olympic events, therefore, laser devices of various kinds will win at least seven or eight gold medals, half a dozen silver, and many bronze—a record that no other class of electronic devices can approach.

LASER APPLICATIONS

To date, the applications of the laser in all fields of scientific measurement have been diverse, extraordinary, and unique. Measurements have been and are being made that simply could not be made in any other fashion. Chemistry, biology, and physics laboratories use many types of lasers to probe, measure, and modify the fundamental properties of matter. Mechanical and aeronautical engineering laboratories are equally well equipped with lasers. For example, laser beams are projected into huge wind tunnels to measure local flow velocity and turbulence.

Lasers are extraordinary tools for identifying materials as well. A medical researcher, by focusing a weak laser beam on an experimental object, can painlessly vaporize a minuscule sample of animal or human tissue for spectroscopic diagnosis of atomic composition, trace elements, and other components. Similarly, an archaeologist can vaporize a tiny sample of a suspect artifact to see if its chemical makeup agrees with its alleged origin.

Outside of pure science and engineering research and development, however, lasers have also been applied in equally diverse and often unanticipated ways in many fields of commerce, manufacturing, industry, and medicine.

Lasers are used in bar code scanners for retail stores, inventory control in warehouses, and supermarket checkout stands. Lasers are found in nearly every elementary surveying instrument these days—for example, lasers mounted on transits are used to obtain contours for leveling of rice paddies and to control dredging barges and automated bulldozers. Laser ranging instruments are used for highway surveying and housing subdivision construction.

In industry, laser beams offer both measuring and manufacturing tools that are flexible and versatile; can be precisely controlled; are well adapted to robotics and numerical control; can be adapted to almost any material or environment; are clean, reliable, and economical to run; and never grow dull.

The simplest industrial applications of high-power lasers come, of course, in the straightforward cutting of materials. Examples include the cutting of armor plate; the cutting of cast iron, without heating or annealing the surrounding material; the cutting of complex patterns in plywood, glass, plastic, or cardboard; and the cutting of cloth for clothing, under computer control, with self-sealing of the fabric edges and minimal waste of material.

But beyond this, there is laser heat treating; laser surface hardening; laser scribing, annealing, deburring, soldering, and resistor trimming; the cutting and repairing of integrated circuits; and the drilling of precise holes in turbine blades (Plate 2), as well as in plastic irrigation pipes and rubber baby bottle nipples.

The laser has also already truly revolutionized the document-scanning, typesetting, newspaper platemaking, and printing industries, at both the high and low ends of the scale. Today, one can print either a newspaper or an interoffice memo with all the information, including the typefaces, stored in a computer memory and printed out by a computer-controlled scanning laser beam. Similar concepts can also be used for the fast and easy marking and labeling of complex mechanical parts made from almost any material. Lasers are now appearing even in consumer products, such as laser video recorders and audio compact disc players.

All of these commercial, industrial, and home applications of laser devices, however diverse and ingenious, thus far have been only preliminary. Indeed, the worldwide sales of laser devices in 1985 totaled only about $400 million–$500 million—or about a quarter of the sales of small computers in the same period by Apple Computers alone.

The worldwide sales of laser systems for all purposes—scientific, engineering, industrial, medical, and military, including ancillary equipment, controls, and materials handling—is believed to have totaled about $4 billion–$5 billion in 1984. Both of these sales figures have been growing annually by 30 percent or more in recent years, although with much higher growth rates in some areas.

In the opinion of most observers, the real boom in the use of lasers in industrial and manufacturing processes is just beginning. For example, large machine tool manufacturers and small laser companies are only now beginning to merge on a wide scale.

Beyond industrial applications, one of the fastest growing areas of laser application is in medicine. Laser surgery is now being used not only to remove skin tumors and conduct other external surgery and to treat many eye diseases but also in ear and throat surgery and gynecology. In addition, using fiber-optic delivery systems, laser surgery is done even inside the intestinal tract and blood vessels.

A form of cancer therapy with lasers is also the subject of much investigation and hope in the medical field. In this therapy, laser light of the proper wavelength activates a photo-sensitive chemical within malignant human tissue, releasing singlet oxygen that destroys the cancer cells.

There are, of course, also many military applications of the laser. Some of the most successful include laser-guided bombs, laser communication links, and laser range finders and aiming devices for guns.

NEW DEVELOPMENTS

Lasers of all types have proved extraordinarily useful devices for bettering the human condition in nearly every area of life, and they will become even more so in future years. But beyond these practical applications, fundamental new basic research advances in the laser field are, even after 25 years, still emerging nearly as rapidly as in the laser's early years.

FREE ELECTRON LASERS

The last few years have seen, for example, the emergence of the so-called free electron laser, in which coherent oscillation at visible or infrared wavelengths is generated by passing the beam from a high-quality electron accelerator through a suitable wave-propagating structure. This device is not really a laser at all, but it is nonetheless a revolutionary development in coherent optical sources whose capabilities are still only in the infant stage.

These devices can provide marvelously tunable, efficient, high-power sources in the far infrared region, from 50 μm out to a few millimeters in wavelength, where laser sources are still somewhat limited. Scientific applications of such sources are manifold; unforeseen industrial applications are equally certain to emerge. The free electron laser may, with further development, also provide a similarly useful source in the visible and ultraviolet regions of the spectrum.

FEMTOSECOND OPTICAL PULSES, BISTABILITY, CHAOS, AND SOLITONS

The incredible advances made in femtosecond laser pulses during the past few years represent one example of progress in the field. Other fundamental developments have also come within the past few years in the basic understanding of new concepts of optical bistability, instabilities, and chaotic optical behavior in lasers. Unexpected developments also occurred in optical solitons and soliton lasers that emerge when such pulses propagate through optical fibers.

TRAPPING AND COOLING OF SINGLE ATOMS AND IONS

Laser researchers are only now succeeding in trapping individual atoms and ions, or small clouds of atoms, and then cooling them to temperatures in the millikelvin range. Once trapped in this fashion, these atoms can be examined and interrogated with laser beams in ways never before possible. This will extend the ultimate precision of physical measurements and laser standards far beyond the few parts in 10^{10} that is now achievable to ultimate accuracies of a few parts in 10^{13} or 10^{14} or even better.

MULTIPLE QUANTUM WELL STRUCTURES

Another fundamental development of the past few years, important for both electronics and lasers, has been the so-called multiple quantum well structures, or artificial layered materials. It has now become possible, using several different techniques such as molecular beam epitaxy or metal-organic chemical vapor deposition, to prepare layered synthetic materials by depositing under precise control a discrete number of atomic layers, first of one material—for example, gallium arsenide—and then another—such as aluminum arsenide—in an alternating sequence.

The result is an essentially perfect artificial crystal with an adjustable period or layer thickness in the range of a few hundred angstroms. Because the properties of the electrons in these multiple quantum well structures can differ greatly from ordinary materials, the electronic and optical properties of these materials offer remarkable new capabilities, including much faster forms of conventional electronic devices.

In optics, the result has already been much more efficient and shorter wavelength diode lasers for use in fiber-optic communications or audio compact disc players, as well as improved photodetectors, light modulators, and other electro-optic devices. By using these diodes as pumps for other laser materials, ultraminiaturized lasers of many different types can be produced.

X-RAY LASERS

Another topic of continuing interest is the extension of laser techniques to the x-ray region. This will always be a difficult task for several reasons, one of which is the difficulty of providing mirrors at these wavelengths. Another basic barrier derives from the fundamental equations of laser theory that say that obtaining laser action becomes more difficult at somewhere between the third and the fifth power of the inverse laser wavelength. Lasers in the x-ray region, if they ever become common, are thus unlikely to be similar to lasers in the optical region.

Nonetheless, Lawrence Livermore Laboratories has recently announced the observation of stimulated emission and laser amplification in the far-ultraviolet or soft x-ray region, at wavelengths of 150–200 Å, in a target plasma pumped by a high-power laser beam. The same lab has also produced a true, if short-lived, one-shot x-ray laser in the few-angstrom region by pumping a suitable laser material directly with a small nuclear explosion.

Given all these recent advances, therefore, it seems clear that the laser field truly is still young, vigorous, and exciting, even as it passes the mature age of 25.

Lasers in Modern Industries

Anthony J. DeMaria

Anthony J. DeMaria

HISTORICAL BACKGROUND

The development of the ammonia beam maser in 1954 ushered in a new breed of active devices that electronic engineers could relate to and use (Gordon et al., 1954). The ammonia beam maser was the first device to use stimulated emission from inverted-population states of quantum mechanical resonances to provide gain for an electromagnetic oscillator. The operation of this quantum mechanical device initiated the field of quantum electronics. In 1984 the field of quantum electronics was 30 years old.

In 1958 Arthur L. Schawlow and Charles H. Townes published a classic paper suggesting the use of the maser principle (with appropriate modification) for the generation of coherent infrared, visible, or ultraviolet radiation (Schawlow and Townes, 1958). The operation of the first ruby laser by Theodore H. Maiman in the latter part of 1960 made available for the first time a visible light beam that had characteristics previously associated only with radio frequency and microwave radiation (Maiman, 1960). The acronym *laser* was formed from *l*ight *a*mplification by *s*timulated *e*mission of *r*adiation. The year 1985 was the 25th anniversary of the laser.

Laser action has now been observed in solids (crystalline and noncrystalline insulators and semiconductors), liquids, gases, and plasmas yielding thousands of discrete wavelengths varying from the vacuum ultraviolet to the millimeter wavelength portion of the electromagnetic spectrum. Dye, color centers, and lead salt lasers now provide tunability over the visible, near-infrared, and infrared spectrum. At present, the abilities of electronic and laser devices overlap for generating radiation in millimeter and submillimeter wavelengths. Scientists are still working toward the generation of coherent radiation at ever-higher frequencies extending to soft and hard x-ray radiation.

Few developments in science have excited the imagination of scientists and engineers as has the laser. The laser made it possible to transport into the optical region all the basic techniques developed for application in the radio and microwave regions, such as harmonic generation; parametric amplification; amplitude, frequency, and phase modulation; homodyne and heterodyne detection; and chirping and pulse compression. In the 25 years since the laser was first realized in the form of pulsed coherent emission from a single ruby crystal, the field has grown at a rate rarely experienced in science. The availability of these intense, coherent optical radiation sources has made it possible for scientists to experiment with optically generated plasmas; optical harmonic generation; stimulated scattering effects; photon echoes; self-induced optical transparency; optical pulses; optical pulse compression; holography; optical shocks; self-trapping of optical radiation; optical parametric amplification; optical ranging to the moon; extremely high resolution spectroscopy; refined measurements of many basic physical properties (length, the speed of light, and so forth); and ultrafast relaxation processes in atoms and molecules.

A MULTIDISCIPLINARY FIELD

Today, the field of laser devices encompasses numerous disciplines. They include solid-state, molecular, and atomic physics; spectroscopy; optics; acoustics; electronics; semiconductor technology; plasma physics; vacuum technology; organic and inorganic chemistry; molecular and atomic kinetics; thin-film technology; glassworking technology; and crystallography. More recently, the field has come to encompass electron-beams, x-rays, fluid dynamics, aerodynamics, and combustion physics. In sum, even without considering applications, the field has grown so fast and proliferated so broadly that scientists are virtually required to specialize within it. As a result, probably no individual today would claim authoritative knowledge over the whole field of laser devices, or even be knowledgeable about most of the significant literature.

THE BIRTH OF THE TECHNOLOGY

During the first 15 years after development of the maser, from approximately 1954 to 1969, the field of quantum electronics was in the technology birth phase. After the operation of the ruby laser in 1960, emphasis shifted from maser to laser devices. This phase was characterized by numerous scientific discoveries and inventions as well as by widely believed visions and predictions of numerous medical, industrial, commercial, scientific, and military applications. During this phase, many laser devices were discovered from a large variety of gases and liquids, as well as from both amorphous and crystalline dielectrics and semiconductor solid-state materials.

Few business opportunities existed during this phase, except to sell components, materials, and devices to researchers concerned with developing the technology base of lasers. Some opportunities were available to sell newly discovered laser sources to researchers interested in probing the linear and nonlinear electromagnetic behavior of atoms and molecules in liquids, solids, and gases. Large corporations were funding in-house research efforts in the technology, as well as capturing significant government research and development contracts. These contracts were directed toward determining the feasibility of numerous military applications during this early development cycle of the technology.

ENGINEERING DEVELOPMENT PHASE

For approximately the next 15 years, laser technology entered the engineering development phase. This phase was characterized by a noticeable decrease in scientific breakthroughs and a perceived impatience with the rate of technological progress toward applications that addressed large markets. This was the period when the statement "the laser is a solution in search of a problem" was often heard. During this phase, many companies with marginal interest in laser technology dropped out of the field. In the same era, entrepreneurs invested considerable effort in searching for markets with large growth potential. In both of these early periods, the military market was larger than the commercial and industrial markets.

MANUFACTURING TECHNOLOGY PHASE

Laser technology has now definitively entered the manufacturing technology phase. Sizable markets have been identified. A strong system and subsystem development effort is in place in which laser devices either significantly lower costs or raise performance leverage over older, more mature technologies. Consequently, product developments have intensified, and many new companies are being created. In addition, large, well-established corporations promote and sell products aimed at markets that laser technology can address uniquely: telecommunications, data processing and storage, entertainment, printing, material working, and medical applications. In contrast to earlier phases, the commercial and industrial markets are now larger than the military market.

Consumers are also beginning to experience laser technology directly through video and audio discs, laser printers for small computers, bar code readers at checkout counters, fiber-optic telecommunications, and various medical treatments. There is evidence of consolidation among numerous small companies oriented toward markets that use laser technology.

NEXT: MATURE TECHNOLOGY PHASE

In the future, laser technology will enter the mature technology, or commodity product, phase, which will be characterized by cost- and volume-driven markets (i.e., economies of scale), requiring capital-intensive manufacturing plants. The laser diode is the first laser device to achieve the mature technology phase. As production volumes and techniques have approached those in the high-volume manufacture of integrated circuits, unit prices of laser diodes have dropped accordingly. Eventually, a few large companies will address the most important laser markets, and chances are good that the surviving manufacturers will not be those known today.

RECENT LASER MARKETS

The dollar value of the 1984 worldwide laser market in the commercial sector and the government and military sector was approximately $2.855 billion and $1.305 billion, respectively, for a total of approximately $4.16 billion (Spectra-Physics Corp., 1983, 1984; DeMaria, 1985). Figure 1 compares the 1983 and 1984 market dollar values. Of the commercial market, approximately $2.502 billion was reported to be in systems and add-ons, whereas laser devices themselves amounted to approximately $353 million of the 1984 world commercial market. As reported in *Lasers and Applications* (1987), "Commercial sales of individual lasers reached $509 million in 1986, up nearly 14%

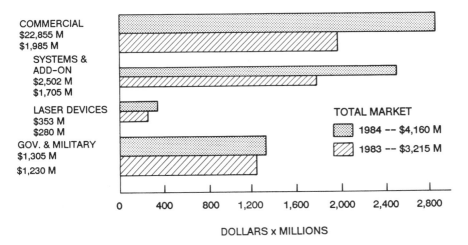

FIGURE 1   Laser industry world markets. SOURCE: Spectra-Physics Corp. (1983, 1984).

over 1985. This year's sales should increase about 10% to $559 million."

From this statement we interpolate that individual laser sales in 1985 totaled approximately $447 million, up approximately 27 percent from the 1984 sales of $353 million. These estimates would lead an entrepreneur rightly to conclude that business opportunities are more plentiful with the inclusion of systems and add-ons in a line of laser devices.

It is important to note in Figure 1 that the military market was smaller than the commercial market in 1983 and 1984. This trend is expected to continue. A 1983 forecast predicted that the worldwide laser market would grow 23 percent annually (Spectra-Physics Corp., 1983, 1984), and that well over 75 laser companies contributed significantly to these world markets. According to *Lasers and Applications* (1987), "Overall, the laser industry continues to grow at double-digit percentage rates. However, the double digits are now in the low teens, not the low twenties as was the case in the early 1980's."

In view of the slow industrial growth in 1986 and 1987, growth of the laser industry in the low teens percentage rate is very respectable. This remarkably high growth rate is comparable to that experienced by the microelectronic and information processing markets.

Figure 2 compares the growth of laser markets in 1984 and 1983. Note that the total market in 1984 grew 29 percent over the 1983 sales. Military sales experienced only a 6 percent

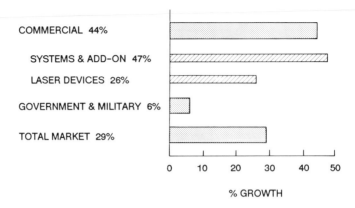

FIGURE 2   Laser industry growth, 1983–1984.

increase in this period, and the commercial market grew by a phenomenally large 44 percent.

COMMERCIAL LASER INDUSTRY

A more detailed look at the 1983 and 1984 commercial laser world market reveals that approximately 63 and 50 percent, respectively, of these 2 years' commercial markets ($1.25 billion and $1.44 billion, respectively) was attributed to printing and graphics associated with information and data processing (see Figure 3). Since Spectra-Physics does not have a product line in the entertainment or computer fields, data on semiconductor lasers and subsystems associated with the video and audio discs and data storage markets were not included in its annual reports (Spectra-Physics Corp., 1983, 1984) and thus are not included in the data shown in Figure 3. The market for audio and video disc entertainment is bringing laser technology directly into the home. *Fortune* forecast that music lovers in the United States would buy 15 million discs in 1985 versus 5.8 million in 1984 (Fortune, 1985). *Fortune* also forecast that sales of players and discs would reach $1.3 billion worldwide in 1985.

The second largest segment of the world's commercial laser market consists of laser material working, which accounted for approximately 11 percent in 1983 ($210 million) and 10 percent in 1984 ($285 million) of the total market. The third largest market segment was communication, which accounted for approximately 8 percent in 1983 and 1984 ($150 million and $225 million, respectively). The medical market is the fourth largest segment, with $105 million in 1983 and $150 million in 1984, capturing just over 5 percent in each of these 2 years. The laser market in metrology, industrial inspection, and science was just under 5 percent in 1983 and 1984 ($90 million and $135 million, respectively) of the total market, and it ranks fifth in size after the medical market. The data capture sector of the market (bar code readers, for example) is the sixth largest in size, with 1983 and 1984 sales of $70 million and $85 million, respectively, and market percentages of just under 4 percent in 1983 and just under 3 percent in 1984. The 1983 numbers include a $35 million miscellaneous category that is not shown as a bar plot in Figure 3 but is included in the $1.986 million total (Spectra-Physics Corp., 1983, 1984).

The expanding applications of lasers in the medical field are a source of great satisfaction to laser researchers. One of the earliest medical applications of lasers was in retina operations. Since then, much progress has been made. Lasers are now being used or investigated for use in cataract surgery, treating bleeding ulcers, opening blocked windpipes, reconnecting severed nerves, removing tumors, and cleaning the plaque that clogs blood vessels. Lasers are also starting to play a role in dermatology, plastic surgery, gynecology, and podiatry (see Rodney C. Perkins in this volume). It is no wonder that the market for laser

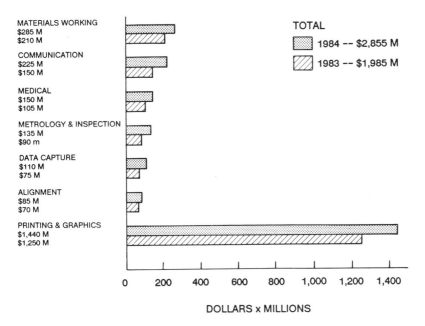

FIGURE 3   Commercial laser industry world market. SOURCE: Spectra-Physics Corp. (1983, 1984).

systems for medical applications is expected to double in each of the next several years. It is an embryonic but fast-growing market.

Figure 4 compares 1984 sales growth with 1983 sales for the market segments identified in Figure 3. The communications market and the metrology and industrial inspection market had an astonishing 50 percent growth in this 2-year period. The data capture and medical sections of the market had outstanding increases of 47 and 43 percent, respectively. The growth of 36 percent achieved by the materials working market and 21 percent by the alignment market would be the envy of most high-technology industries. The printing and graphics segment of the laser market had the smallest growth—15 percent—of the identified market.

In the automated offices of tomorrow, it has been widely forecast that video screens will replace ink and paper. Today, however, office automation is producing more rather than less paper. The printers that help computers create much of this paper have become a $2.4 billion industry, with the promise that printer sales will more than double before the decade ends (The Wall Street Journal, 1984). Semiconductor laser printer technology is expected to become the major competitor against ink jet printers in the future computer printer market. One or both of

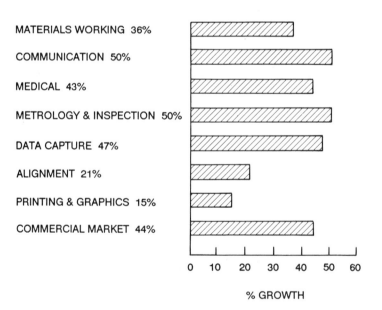

FIGURE 4   Commercial laser industry growth, 1983–1984.

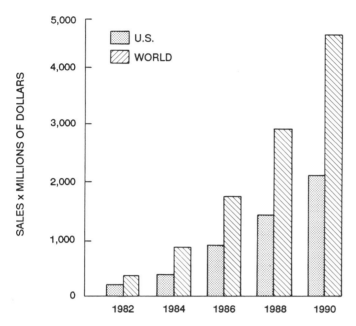

FIGURE 5   Fiber optics market: fibers, cables, transceivers, components.
SOURCE: Business Week (1984).

these technologies is expected to displace the typewriter technology used today.

Much of the laser communications market—that is, the fiber
optics telecommunications market—is held by large, vertically
integrated corporations such as AT&T, ITT, and Nippon
Telegraph & Telephone and is thus not available to other
manufacturers. Undoubtedly, this accounts for the relatively
small fraction of the total world market of the commercial laser
industry attributable to the laser communications market, as
shown in Figure 3. By 1990 the fiber optics world market is
expected to exceed $4.5 billion per year, whereas the U.S.
market will be approximately $2 billion per year (Figure 5).
Business Week has predicted that the end of conventional copper
wire in the telecommunications industry could come as early as
the turn of the century; moreover, semiconductor lasers coupled with fiber optics technology will make ground and undersea cable communication so inexpensive that few commercial
communication satellites will be launched in the 1990s (Business
Week, 1984). There were 250,000 miles of optical telecommunication fibers installed in the United States in 1983. Northern

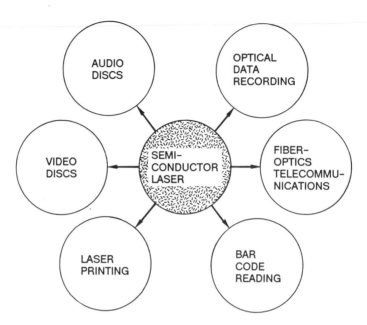

FIGURE 6   Applications of semiconductor lasers.

Business Information, Inc., forecast that approximately 1.3 million miles of telecommunication fiber would be installed in the United States in 1986. This installation is expected to increase to 4.5 million miles in 1990 (Business Week, 1984). The development of laser communications technology is discussed in detail by C. K. N. Patel later in this volume.

Over the last 20 years, three areas of laser technology have received continuous and extensive research and development support: laser weapons, controlled fusion, and semiconductor laser development. By most estimates, the practical realization of the first two is still believed to be 20 years away. Because of their importance to national security and economic well-being, they have received extensive government research and development support in many countries. The semiconductor laser, on the other hand, has been developed primarily with industrial research and development funds. This development has spawned many new sectors of major industries, such as telecommunications, printing, video and audio discs, data recording, and bar code reading (Figure 6). In another example of the large markets generated by semiconductor lasers, Frost & Sullivan, Inc. (1986), has projected tremendous market growth over the next few years for optical disc system manufacturers and retailers for personal computers. They have forecast a market of $2.5 billion in 1990 for optical disc systems.

Optical discs can offer much greater information density than current magnetic storage devices at a lower cost per byte. Consequently, they are expected to generate the next revolution in mass storage. The technologies for write-once and read-only optical discs have been well established for some time. They use a modulated laser beam to permanently engrave a submicron-size bubble or pit in the active layer of a medium. Intensive research has been focused on erasable optical discs using a semiconductor laser that causes either a phase change or magneto-optical change in a medium. Compact disc read-only memories store 550 megabytes of data that cannot be altered or erased and were the first to reach the market. Write-once discs are relatively new to the market and typically hold 1–2 gigabytes and let users store and update information without eliminating data already stored on the disc. Erasable discs are not expected to appear until 1988 and will permit continual reuse.

The success of the semiconductor diode laser in bringing about many new sectors of major industries is probably attributable to its compatibility with semiconductor integrated circuits. Its small size, low manufacturing cost, low voltage and power requirements, and high efficiency make it compatible with modern electronic technology. The semiconductor laser is the first truly mass-produced laser. It has been reported that Mitsubishi Electronic Corporation produced 400,000 semiconductor lasers monthly in 1985. It is expected that 10 million diode lasers will be sold in 1987, with the vast majority going into audio disc players and low-cost printers. Laser diode production has become a commodity process with commodity pricing strategies.

PHOTONICS VERSUS ELECTRONICS

In the early days of electronics, vacuum tubes played an important role in developing the industrial base of the radio frequency, microwave, and millimeter wave portion of the electromagnetic spectrum. Similarly, gas lasers and optically pumped solid-state lasers have been important in developing the industrial base of lightwave technology in the new field of quantum electronics. There is also a clear analogy between the roles played by the semiconductor diode laser and the transistor in establishing the industrial base of their respective spectral re-

LANDMARKS IN ELECTRONICS

The field of electronics began in 1883 when Thomas Edison discovered, while working with his carbon filament lamp, that current flowed across a vacuum when he placed a positive voltage on a metal plate a small distance from a glowing carbon filament in a vacuum envelope. This phenomenon was the basis of all electron tubes, which were the foundation of electronics until the era of the transistor began in 1949. From 1883 to 1904, no one exploited the effect to make a useful device for detecting, generating, and amplifying electrical signals, even though the telephone industry during that era could have benefited from the invention of a suitable amplifier. In 1887 Heinrich Hertz transmitted and received radio signals within his laboratory and experimentally confirmed James Clerk Maxwell's equations, which had been published in 1864. In 1901 Guglielmo Marconi propagated radio waves across the Atlantic Ocean from Poldhu, Cornwall, England, to St. John, Newfoundland, Canada, without the aid of electronic amplifiers and oscillators. The vacuum diode rectifier was invented by John Ambrose Fleming in 1904. The famous audion, the three-element vacuum tube, was invented by Lee de Forest in 1906 and was the first electronic amplifier. Just 29 years after Edison's discovery in 1883, the first electronic oscillator came into being in 1912 with Edwin Armstrong's invention of the regenerative circuit and operation of the first coherent electronic oscillator. From that point on, the electronics industry developed rapidly, heralding the beginning of radio and modern electronics.

gions. At present, the technologies of integrated optics and guided wave optics are being developed by researchers whose goal is to obtain benefits in the optical region similar to those obtained earlier in the electronic region by planar electronic integrated circuits, hybrid circuits, and planar microwave/millimeter strip-line technologies. The ability to realize both optical and electronic devices from compound semiconductor technology is largely responsible for the present intensive research on compound semiconductors.

The field of electronics was created with the invention of the vacuum tube around the turn of this century. The heart of electronic technology is the device that controls the flow of an electron stream (electrical current) either in a vacuum (the vacuum tube) or in a solid (the transistor). Since the laser controls the flow of a photon stream (light), the laser can be considered the heart of quantum electronics technology. This analogy can be carried one step further by including in the new term *photonics* the field of quantum electronics, which includes lasers, as well as optoelectronics, electro-optics, acousto-optics, fiber optics, integrated optics, and nonlinear optics. One should not jump to the conclusion that electronics and photonics technologies compete against each other. Rather, these two fields are complementary. Photonics depends heavily on electronics technology, and is useful for those tasks that cannot be performed using electronics technology. By performing such tasks, photonics creates new segments of existing industries, thereby establishing a niche for itself and also further expanding the base of electronic technology.

How much time will be required to commercialize the field of photonics? Indications are that electronics developed slowly during its earlier phase and then more rapidly in later stages. Photonics, in contrast, developed more rapidly during its earlier phase because of the technical support provided by the field of electronics and is expected to continue its swift progress. As photonics continues its rapid expansion past its 25th birthday, it is also expanding the future horizons of electronics technology.

Since the 1912 invention of the electronic oscillator, there has been a steady drive toward the production and use of coherent electromagnetic energy of higher and higher frequencies. This tendency results partly from the realization that an increase in transmitted information, directivity, and efficiency can be achieved by increasing carrier frequency and partly from the crowding and interference between existing frequency bands. Another important push toward generating coherent radiation of higher frequencies resulted from researchers' interest in using these waves to probe atoms in solids, liquids, and gases by employing experimental techniques such as nuclear magnetic resonance, paramagnetic resonance, and cyclotron resonance. To meet these needs, investigators have devised active electronic devices that use the flow of an electron stream in a vacuum or the flow of electrons and holes in semiconductor materials. They have been greatly improved for the generation of higher frequencies. Examples of such devices are vacuum tubes, transistors, magnetrons, klystrons, traveling wave tubes, parametric amplifiers, and tunnel diodes. With these devices, researchers have generated coherent radiation in the hundreds of gigahertz. With the use of harmonic generators, this figure has been extended by approximately one order of magnitude. Almost without exception, as soon as higher frequency devices become available, researchers rush to use them in probing the atomic and molecular domain of liquids, gases, and solids.

The physical dimensions of the resonators used to select the oscillating frequency of conventional oscillators in the higher frequency range are of the order of magnitude of the wavelength of the radiation generated. As a result, it becomes extremely difficult to construct resonators to the small dimensions required at submillimeter wavelengths. In the late 1940s and early 1950s, it became apparent to workers in the field that it was becoming impossible to apply the old methods of scaling down existing devices for higher frequency generations. In the search for alternate methods, researchers came to realize that natural resonators in the form of atomic and molecular systems could be used to amplify and even generate coherent electromagnetic energy. This realization led to the invention of the ammonia beam maser and the laser and to the creation of the field of photonics.

SELECTED INDUSTRIAL APPLICATIONS

This section will briefly discuss selected applications of lasers in semiconductor integrated circuits manufacturing, radar systems, material cutting and drilling, and inspection of electric power cables. These examples indicate the breadth of laser applications in modern industries, such as microelectronics, avionics, machining, and electric power.

MANUFACTURING SEMICONDUCTOR INTEGRATED CIRCUITS

The technology of semiconductor integrated circuits has contributed greatly to the electronic, or information, revolution which may hold more enduring implications for mankind than the industrial revolution (Abelson and Hammond, 1977). Of the large number of different integrated circuits now produced, the dynamic random access memory (DRAM) chips have the largest unit sales and volume and the greatest dependency on the manufacturing learning curve for reducing costs and increasing yields to meet the aggressive pricing strategy of competitors. DRAM chips use the most advanced processing technologies to achieve the highest density of semiconductor devices per chip. They also have one of the shortest product life cycles in the semiconductor industry; the last 25 years have seen a rapid increase in the complexity of these chips, from the first 4-kilobit (K) product up through the 16K, 64K, 256K, and the present

1-megabit DRAM chip. The rate of progress has been breath-taking from the standpoint of the number of chips per wafer, the rapidly decreasing layout rules down to the present micron to submicron dimensions, increasing die sizes, decreasing number of dies per wafer, and increasing capital cost for a wafer fabrication factory. Consequently, a manufacturer's ability to be the first to market and to increase sharply chip yields early in the production cycle can usually determine success or failure in the market. Because of the insatiable appetite of computer manufacturers for an ever-larger memory capacity per chip, fierce competition is now under way to be the first to market with 4- and 16-megabit DRAM products.

Laser technology has made it possible for manufacturers of DRAM chips to increase their yield and volume dramatically in the early phases of their production cycle by use of a technique often referred to as laser redundancy (Posa, 1981; Smith, 1981). Laser redundancy enables manufacturers to design spare, normally inactive, address encoders into their memory chips. When a portion of a memory chip is found not to meet specifications during initial die testing, a pulsed 1.06-μm laser with neodymium ions in yttrium-aluminum garnet (Nd^{3+}:YAG) is used to "explode" away the polysilicon conductor connecting the encoder addressing that portion of the circuitry, thereby disconnecting the defective portion from the circuit. The laser system is then used to open the polysilicon conductor, shorting out the spare address encoder and thereby connecting that encoder to the other circuitry of the chip.

Figure 7a shows a small portion of an integrated circuit, including functioning polysilicon film conductor interconnecting lines, crystal silicon substrate, silicon dioxide insulator film, and aluminum film interconnecting lines. Figure 7b shows a polysilicon film interconnect line cut with a laser. Because the polysilicon has a higher absorption coefficient for the laser radiation than the crystal silicon, it melts selectively and evaporates under high-intensity, pulsed, 1.06-μm laser irradiation.

The use of laser redundancy in the manufacture of 64K DRAM chips typically increased yields by 2 to 3 times during the start-up phase of manufacturing and led to an average 40–50 percent improvement in the number of good dies produced per wafer in the start-up phase. Manufacturers have been able to obtain an equivalent number of chips from one manufacturing facility as they previously obtained from two facilities.

Mostek Corporation was one of the early users of laser redundancy in the manufacturing of 64K DRAMs. It took Mostek 1.5 years to produce 2 million 4K DRAM chips during the start-up phase when they introduced that product to the market in the early 1970s. Because of the added complexity of the 16K DRAM chip, it

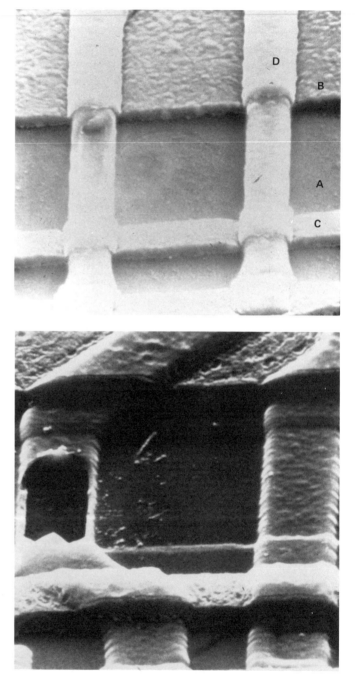

FIGURE 7   Top: Small portions of an integrated circuit showing the single-crystal silicon substrate (A), the silicon dioxide insulator film (B), the aluminum film interconnecting conductor lines (C), and the polysilicon film interconnecting conductor lines (D). Bottom: A polysilicon film interconnecting conductor line cut with a laser.

took Mostek 2 years to reach the 2-million-chip production level. The process took only about 9 months for the 64K DRAM chips because of the use of laser redundancy. Based on this outstanding Mostek result, laser redundancy techniques are now used extensively in the manufacture of complex semiconductor chips.

LASER MATERIAL WORKING

The ability of a laser to deliver a high-intensity beam of radiation through the atmosphere and heat an absorbing material has drawn attention to its use in the material-working industry for such applications as cutting, drilling, welding, heat treating, and melting. The utility of the laser in these applications can be seen by referring to the Stefan-Boltzmann law of radiation: The total energy radiated per unit area by a perfect thermal source is equal to the fourth power of the temperature times the Stefan-Boltzmann radiation constant. For instance, a power density of 1 million W/cm^2 corresponds to a thermal source operating at 20,500 K. By means of optical focusing, the laser can easily achieve temperatures in this range and is therefore capable of providing such high energy concentrations that its focused radiation can melt or vaporize any known material.

Figure 8 shows the laser radiation power density and the

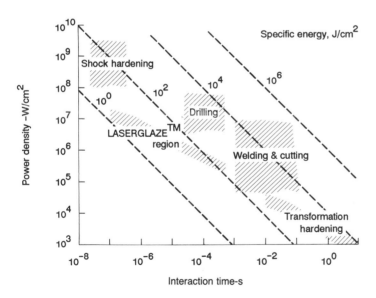

FIGURE 8   Laser beam-material interaction spectrum. Laser power density (W/cm^2) and material interaction time (s) required by various material-working tasks.

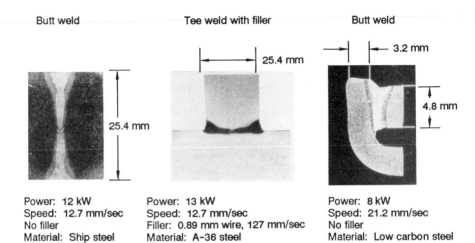

Butt weld	Tee weld with filler	Butt weld

25.4 mm

25.4 mm

3.2 mm

4.8 mm

Power: 12 kW
Speed: 12.7 mm/sec
No filler
Material: Ship steel

Power: 13 kW
Speed: 12.7 mm/sec
Filler: 0.89 mm wire, 127 mm/sec
Material: A–36 steel

Power: 8 kW
Speed: 21.2 mm/sec
No filler
Material: Low carbon steel

FIGURE 9   Typical weld configurations performed with a CO_2 laser under the conditions indicated.

interaction time of the radiation with a material required to accomplish various important material-processing tasks (Banas and Webb, 1982). For a laser beam moving continuously across a material, the interaction time can be defined as the time required for the incident laser spot to move one diameter relative to the surface of the workpiece. For a material process requiring short pulses of laser radiation, the interaction time is the duration of the pulse, since the material can be assumed to be stationary during the short irradiation process.

Figure 9 shows three typical laser welds performed with carbon dioxide (CO_2) lasers (Duhamel and Banas, 1983). A three-stage, gas-recirculating, closed-cycle, electric-discharge CO_2 laser can yield 9–12 kW of continuous output power. The use of fast gas-flowing techniques to achieve several tens of kilowatts of continuous power from electrically excited CO_2 lasers (DeMaria, 1973) has been responsible for placing CO_2 lasers in a dominant position for large material-working applications. In the next decade, laser material processing in manufacturing is expected to increase dramatically. The Nd^{3+}:YAG, ruby, Nd^{3+}:glass, and CO_2 lasers are expected to be the most widely used in these applications.

LASER RADAR

Laser radar technology is an obvious progression of radar technology from the radio frequency, microwave, and millimeter wave region of the spectrum into the optical region (i.e., infrared, visible, near ultraviolet). Laser radar technology has both advantages and disadvantages when compared with conventional radar technology. Consequently, laser radar systems will complement and not compete with conventional, lower frequency radar systems. Laser radar systems will be used predominantly in those applications that cannot be addressed by conventional radar systems.

Range finders are the most basic radar systems of either the microwave or the laser variety. They measure the range to a target by measuring the time of flight of a transmitted and an echo pulse of electromagnetic radiation. The speed of the target can be obtained by measuring the change in range as a function of time. Range finders can also provide information about the azimuth to a target. Radars of this kind are known as incoherent radar systems.

Coherent radar systems are more complex and have the ability to measure the velocity of the targets by means of the Doppler effect. This type of radar was originally used extensively in the early development of radar technology to detect moving targets against stationary background clutter. Coherent radar systems measure the Doppler shift of the echo radiation by comparing the frequency of the received echo signal with the frequency of the transmitted radiation. This comparison is accomplished by heterodyning, or mixing, the returned signal with the signal of the system's frequency reference (called the local oscillator) on a detector. By maintaining the frequency of the transmitter signal either above or below the local oscillator signal by a fixed value determined by electronic control circuits, and superimposing on the detector the local oscillator signal with the return signal from a stationary target, an interference pattern that modulates the amplitude of the detected laser radiation is generated on the detector. This "beat" signal is equal to the difference between the frequencies of the transmitted and local oscillator signals. Since this beat signal is arranged to occur within the radio frequency range (tens to hundreds of megahertz), electronic amplifiers tuned to this frequency can process the signal electronically and obtain the same signal-to-noise benefits well known in conventional heterodyne radio receivers. Measurement of the deviation of this known beat signal by the Doppler effect caused by the moving target provides a measurement of the speed of the target.

An additional advantage of the coherent radar system is that one can increase the power of the local oscillator signal on the detector to achieve the theoretical detector performance, which is the quantum noise-limited sensitivity. A laser radar, using CO_2 lasers, typically operates in the 10.6-μm wavelength region

(Silverman, 1982). At this wavelength, HgCdTe detectors at present provide the optimum sensitivity. A figure of merit for detectors is usually given in terms of noise-equivalent power, or NEP. Heterodyne NEPs of 2×10^{-19}, 5×10^{-18}, and 2×10^{-17} WHz have been measured with HgCdTe detectors operating at 1 GHz at 77 K, 195 K, and 300 K, respectively.

Table 1 compares some of the relevant parameters of x-band and CO_2 laser radars. The laser radar operates at a frequency 3,000 times higher (or at a wavelength 3,000 times shorter) than an x-band radar. The large difference in wavelengths between the CO_2 laser radar and the x-band radar results in large differences in reflection characteristics of targets for the two technologies. Variation in target surface dimensions (i.e., surface roughness) typically are greater than the wavelengths of CO_2 laser radars, but less than the wavelengths of x-band radars. Since man-made targets usually have smoother surfaces than natural targets, even small man-made targets such as wires have a larger cross-section than natural targets for laser radars. Figure 10 shows the ratio of detector signal current to noise current (i_s/i_n) as a function of range for various natural and man-made targets irradiated with a pulsed, coherent CO_2 laser radar system having 400 mW of average power and an HgCdTe detector.

TABLE 1   Comparison of Basic Radar Parameters

Radar Characteristic	CO_2 Laser Radar	x-Band Radar
Frequency, Hz	3×10^{13}	10^{10}
Wavelength, cm	10^{-3}	3
Beamwidth, λ/D, radians	10^{-3}/dia.	3/dia.
Doppler sensitivity, $2v/\lambda$, Hz	2,000 × velocity	2/3 × velocity
Photon energy, Joules	2×10^{-20}	6.6×10^{-24}

Note: $D=$ diameter, in cm; v = velocity, in cm/s.

Since the beam divergence varies directly with wavelength and indirectly with transmitting aperture, CO_2 laser radars have 3,000 times smaller beam divergence than x-band radars with the same aperture. Since the Doppler shift varies inversely with wavelength, the CO_2 laser radar has three orders of magnitude higher Doppler sensitivity than an x-band radar (see Figure 11). Figure 11 shows, for instance, that for a radar frequency of 30 THz (CO_2 laser frequency), a target moving at 0.5 km/h (about 1/10 the speed of a person walking) yields a Doppler signal of 100 kHz, whereas a 30-GHz microwave radar would yield a Doppler signal of 0.1 kHz.

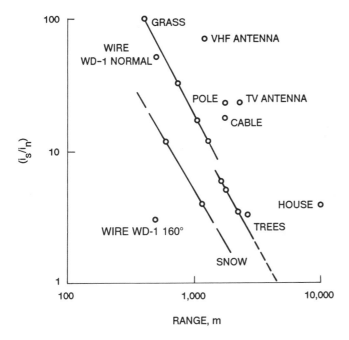

FIGURE 10   Signal-to-noise ratio of a CO_2 laser radar (400 mW average power, 75 W peak power) for various natural and man-made targets.

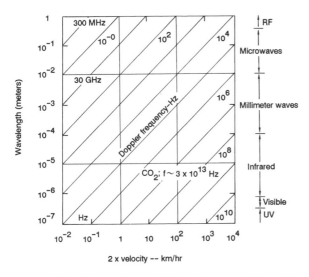

FIGURE 11   Comparison of Doppler sensitivity: Doppler frequency shift as a function of radar wavelength and target velocity.

Since the photon energy of the CO_2 laser radar is 3,000 times higher than that of the x-band radar, the laser radar beam has 3,000 times fewer photons per unit of energy than the x-band radar. If one photon in unit time is the minimum detectable signal, then the operation of a CO_2 laser radar is limited to a smaller field of view than the x-band radar for the same transmitted power. Consequently, the laser radar is not suited to wide-area search applications, but is well suited to applications requiring ultrahigh sensitivity in range, azimuth, Doppler shift, image resolution, and small field of view.

It is important to point out that laser radar suffers from poorer propagation characteristics through the atmosphere than conventional microwave radar because of higher back-scatter from rain, snow, haze, and fog and because of higher absorption by water in the atmosphere. Consequently, in the earth's atmosphere, laser radars have a shorter range than microwave radars. Fortunately, the operating wavelengths of CO_2 lasers falls within one of the best atmospheric windows when compared with other laser wavelengths. Consequently, for applications in the atmosphere, the relatively long wavelength of 10.6 μm for CO_2 lasers over other lasers, such as Nd^{3+}:YAG, ruby, and semiconductor lasers, makes the CO_2 laser radar the system of choice for most applications.

Figure 12 shows general areas of applications of various radar technologies. *Ladar* is a commonly used acronym for "laser radar," and was formed from *la*ser *d*etection *a*nd *r*anging following the example of the word *radar,* which was originally an acronym formed from *ra*dio *d*etection *a*nd *r*anging. (*Lidar, l*ight *d*etection *a*nd *r*anging, is also used.)

Figure 13 compares a telescopic photograph of a control tower at a range of 1.2 km with an image taken by a 15-year-old coherent CO_2 laser radar. The ladar system used a binary (black and white) gray scale and was not intended to produce a photographic-quality image. The output power of the early ladar used to produce this image was 0.25 W at a pulse repetition rate of 30,000 pulses/s. The trees in the far background of the scene do not show up in the laser radar image because of a range-gating technique used by the ladar system. The evergreen trees at the bottom of the photograph do show up in the ladar image because their return signals fell within the time window of the time-gated receiver. Since glass is absorbing at 10.6 μm, the windows appear black in the ladar image. The antennas on top of the control tower are difficult to see against the sky in the photograph but are easily visible in the laser radar image. The ability of CO_2 ladars to detect small obstacles such as wires,

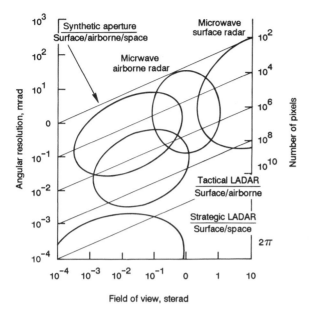

FIGURE 12   Active sensors capabilities: general areas of applications of various radar technologies from an angular resolution and field-of-view perspective.

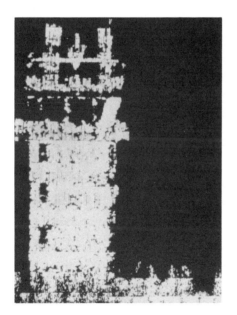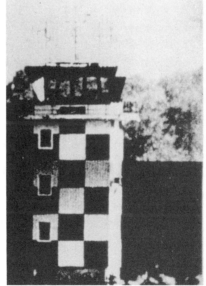

FIGURE 13   Comparison of a photographic image (taken through a telescope) with a black-and-white binary scale CO_2 coherent laser radar composite image. The trees in the far background were not recorded in the radar image because of range-gating techniques used in the ladar system. Range: 1,200 m; average power: ¼ W; pulse rate: 30,000/s.

poles, and antennas makes them ideally suited for obstacle and terrain avoidance applications in helicopters. They are also compatible with the 8- to 12-μm passive night-viewing avionic systems now in use.

One of the most exciting potential applications of ladar is in the measurement of wind velocities in the upper atmosphere by measuring, from the space shuttle, the Doppler shift from backscatter off naturally occurring aerosols in the upper atmosphere. The operation of such a system is expected to improve greatly the accuracy of weather forecasting.

ELECTRIC CABLE INSPECTION

When it was established that polyethylene (PE) and cross-linked PE (XLPE) material had intrinsically high dielectric strengths, on the order of 800 kV/mm, the electric power industry expected 40-year lifetimes for underground electric power cables in distribution systems using such materials. Consequently, in the 1960s, the electric power industry began to make extensive use of underground cables using PE and XLPE as the dielectric between the inner and outer conductors. The expected lifetime was not achieved even at average stress levels of 2–4 kV/mm, even though such stress levels provided 200–400 times smaller voltage gradients than the intrinsic dielectric strength of the material. The failure rate for cables put into service since the 1960s reached a level that disturbed the electric power industry. It led the Electric Power Research Institute, the U.S. Department of Energy, and cable manufacturers to launch a research and development program in the 1970s to solve the problem of the premature failures of PE and XLPE cables.

The cables are produced in a continuous operation. A central conductor of stranded copper wire passes through an extruder that coats it with a smooth, thin semiconducting shield consisting of PE filled with carbon black. Over this opaque semiconducting surface, the white PE insulation is extruded and then cross-linked with heat, ultraviolet radiation, or electron bombardment. A second semiconducting shield of PE and carbon black is then extruded over the insulation, followed by a mesh of stranded copper wires and finally a protective plastic coating.

The research and development programs indicated that the aging of the insulation generates branched channels caused by dielectric breakdown, which in turn causes an electrical short circuit between the outer ground conductor and the inner conductor (see Figure 14). The branched channel structure, or "trees," of dielectric breakdown in the insulation is believed to be

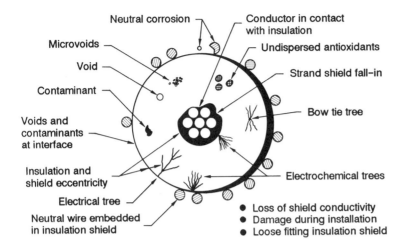

FIGURE 14   Common causes of electric power cable failures.

caused by surface imperfections at interfaces within the cable and by irregularities in the insulating materials. These irregularities are caused by gas- or vapor-filled voids, contaminating particles, inhomogeneous variation of density in the materials, and other defects. Unfortunately, visual inspection is not possible during the manufacturing process, where these defects arise, because PE is normally a milky white, opaque material except when immersed in hot oil.

Corona testing is a nondestructive inspection technique that can detect 50-μm-diameter voids in 500-ft lengths of cable. The disadvantage of the technique is that it cannot detect contaminants and flaws, voids filled with liquids or vapors, and microvoids 1–10 μm in diameter. The technique also does not provide on-line inspection during the manufacturing process, nor can it locate the position of the defect.

The inspection procedure now commonly used is to cut out a 2-in. piece of manufactured cable every 10,000 ft, slice it into 0.5-in. portions, slice these portions into 0.020-in. wafers, make these wafers transparent by immersing them in hot oil, and then inspect the wafers visually under a 15-power microscope. The obvious disadvantages of this technique are that it is neither an on-line, real-time inspection process nor a nondestructive procedure.

One promising approach to an on-line, real-time technique for nondestructive inspection of cable is based on the fact that PE and XLPE are almost transparent in the far infrared.

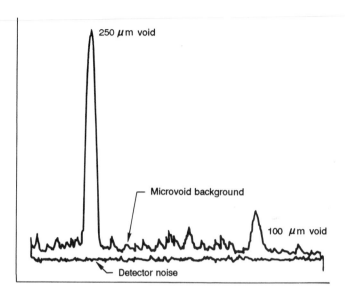

FIGURE 15   Signals of a far-infrared laser inspection system from voids in cross-linked polyethylene insulation used in electric power distribution cable (25 KV moving cable).

Investigation of lasers that emit radiation in the far infrared (Chang et al., 1970) led to a nondestructive technique for continuously monitoring the quality of electric power cables in real time (Cantor et al., 1981). A monitoring system based on this technique scans around the cable before the outer ground conductor and its protective coating are extruded onto the cable. The laser radiation scattered by voids, contaminants, or other defects in the dielectric is collected and detected, and its magnitude is digitally recorded. The speed of the cable through the system is monitored to maintain a complete record of signal amplitude caused by the scattered radiation as a function of cable position. Figure 15 shows typical signals obtained at a 118-μm laser wavelength and 0.1-W laser power with a germanium-doped silicon detector cooled with liquid helium. Figure 16 shows an experimental arrangement of such a system. It is important to note that because of the long laser wavelength (submillimeter wavelengths), the mirrors are fabricated from finely machined aluminum and do not require extensive polishing.

It is too early to determine the practical effect of laser inspection in the manufacture of electrical power cable, but it is already apparent that the technology will provide useful research instrumentation for the industry.

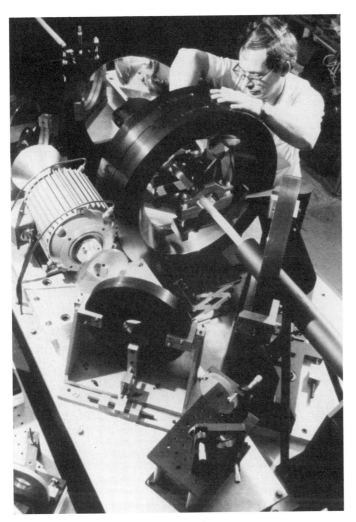

FIGURE 16 Optics used in a far-infrared laser inspection system for electric power cable insulation.

CONCLUSIONS

Laser technology is young and robust, with a highly promising and exciting future. It is now spawning new products and opening major new segments of basic industries that will ensure its growth well into the next century. The fields of fiber-optic telecommunications, optical audio and video discs, optical data storage, optoelectronics, lasers for material working (cutting, welding, heat treating, hole drilling, and scribing), laser applications in medicine, laser instrumentation, and military applications are still in their infancy; thus, considerable growth is yet to come.

The most serious challenge in laser technology is the continuing shortage of photonic engineers required to develop the numerous new and rapidly evolving products the technology is generating, to continually advance the state of the art required to meet new product needs, and to work at the interface between electronics and photonics technologies. An engineer in this field needs a background in optics and electronics and in quantum electronics. Most engineers working in the field today are either physicists who have learned some electronics or electronic engineers who have learned some optics. The offering of a formal undergraduate engineering curriculum in photonic engineering would be a big boost to this important emerging field of technology.

REFERENCES

Abelson, P. H., and A. L. Hammond. 1977. Science 195(4283):1085.

Banas, C. M., and R. Webb. 1982. Proc. IEEE 70(June):556.

Business Week. May 21, 1984. 181.

Cantor, A. J., P. K. Cheo, M. C. Foster, and L. A. Newman. 1981. IEEE J. Quantum Electron. QE-17(April):477–489.

Chang, T. Y., T. J. Bridges, and E. G. Burkhardt. 1970. Appl. Phys. Lett. 17(Sept. 15):249–251.

DeMaria, A. J. 1973. Proc. IEEE 61(June):731–748.

DeMaria, A. J. 1985. Optics News 10:15.

Duhamel, P. F., and C. M. Banas. 1983. 1983 ASM Conference on Applications of Lasers in Material Processing, Los Angeles, 24–26 January. Reprint 8301-020. Metals Park, Ohio: American Society of Metals.

Frost & Sullivan, Inc. 1986. PC Optical Disk Market in the U.S. New York: Frost & Sullivan, Inc.

Fortune. July 8, 1985. 104.

Gordon, J. P., H. J. Zeiger, and C. H. Townes. 1954. Phys. Rev. 95:282.

Lasers and Applications. January 1987. 65.

Maiman, T. H. 1960. Phys. Rev. Lett. 4:564.

Posa, J. G. 1981. Electronics 28(July):117–120.

Schawlow, A. L., and C. H. Townes. 1958. Phys. Rev. 112:1940.

Silverman, B. B. 1982. Proc. IEEE 1982 National Aerospace and Electronics Conf. 2:568–575.

Smith, R. T. 1981. Electronics 28(July):131–134.

Spectra-Physics Corp. 1983. Annual Report. Spectra-Physics, Inc., San Jose, Calif.

Spectra-Physics Corp. 1984. Annual Report. Spectra-Physics, Inc., San Jose, Calif.

The Wall Street Journal. March 16, 1984. 29.

Lasers in Communications and Information Processing

C. Kumar N. Patel

Since the invention of the laser in 1958, a tremendous amount of progress has been made in the field, both in the science and technology of lasers themselves and in the variety of applications of lasers (Schawlow and Townes, 1958). Lasers now cover the range of wavelengths from x rays to microwaves, where they merge with other coherent-radiation sources, such as klystrons. Uses of lasers also cover a broad spectrum: science, remote sensing, monitoring, detection, information transmission and processing, industrial processing, defense, and medicine and surgery.

In some fields, the introduction of lasers may be heralded as a "killer" technology that totally displaces an existing technology; in other fields, it may be a new-domain technology that has uncovered applications not thought of before; in still other fields, laser technology may turn out to fill a niche not occupied by any other technology. As John S. Mayo of AT&T Bell Laboratories has pointed out, the transistor should be considered a killer technology because it displaced vacuum tubes (Mayo, 1985); automatic speech recognition appears to be a new-domain technology; broadcast television ought to be viewed as occupying a niche in the information dissemination world without significantly changing the quality of information and coexisting with radio, newspapers, and other means of disseminating information. It is too early to decide how lasers will fit into various fields. This paper will describe accomplishments and future possibilities in communications and information processing and will allow the reader to decide how laser technology will shape the existing technologies. What remains to be seen is whether lasers have contributed to a revolution or are part of the gradual evolution of the information age.

Society relies on at least three distinct activities in the information age. The first is the creation of information; the second is the transmission of information; and the third is the manipulation of information. This paper will focus on accomplished and anticipated changes brought about by the exploitation of lasers and associated technology in information transmission and processing. These two areas share many properties but have many significant differences as well.

LASERS IN COMMUNICATIONS

The explosion in the use of lasers in communications has come about through a simultaneous improvement in the quality of the medium through which light energy is transmitted and the increased understanding of the laser sources, detectors, and associated phenomena that allow tailoring of the properties of materials and devices. For economic exploitation of fiber-based lightwave systems for information transmission, two parameters, sometimes combined, are very important. The first is the maximum data transmission rate, which itself is limited by capabilities of the lasers, detectors, and associated electronics. The second is the maximum distance a bit stream can be transmitted over an optical fiber before a repeater is necessary. It is clear that the properties of the optical fiber contribute to the second parameter. Relevant optical fiber properties are the absorption losses and the chromatic dispersion. An appropriate standard of measurement for an information transmission system is the product of bit rate and distance, that is, the distance between repeaters at a prescribed bit rate. The impact of lightwaves on the capacity of a communication system is summarized in Figure 1, which shows the growth in system capacity since the construction of the first telephone lines in 1890. The introduction of lightwave systems is causing a sharp change in the rate at which channel capacity has increased over the past 100 years.

OPTICAL FIBERS

Free space propagation never caught on for terrestrial lightwave communications because of the potentional interruptions arising from fog, rain, and other natural phenomena. Lightwave transmission through guided media, optical fibers, is not a new

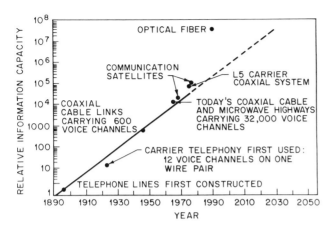

FIGURE 1   Channel capacity improvement as a function of time. Note the discontinuous change in the average slope with the introduction of lightwave systems.

phenomenon, but the use of fibers for lightwave communications puts stringent requirements on the tolerable losses in the medium. More than 20 years ago, Kao and Hochkam (1966) proposed the use of clad glass fiber as a lightwave transmission medium. Initially, materials limitation due to absorption of impurities led to transmission losses of more than 100 dB/km in the 1960s. By the early 1970s, fiber losses were reduced to about 10 dB/km at 850 nm in silica fibers (see Figure 2) (S. R. Nagel, personal communication). Much of the improvement was brought about by a careful elimination of impurities. These losses were low enough that the early lightwave systems were designed to operate in the low-loss region of 850 nm (Figure 2) and use the available GaAs-GaAlAs heterostructure lasers.

The next decade saw a continued elimination of impurities, such as OH. By 1976 this resulted in optical fibers with losses as small as 1.0 dB/km at 1.3 μm (Figure 2). The next generation of lightwave systems was designed to take advantage of the low-loss region near 1.3 μm. This also has the additional advantage of being a region where the fiber dispersion is zero. Further improvements in fibers arose from reductions in OH and have shifted the minimum loss region to 1.55 μm (Figure 2), where the losses are 0.15 dB/km (Nelson et al., 1985). The current generation of lightwave systems is designed to take advantage of these low losses. See Appendix A for a detailed discussion of fiber loss and dispersion as they affect lightwave communications.

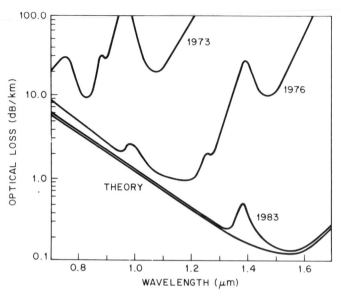

FIGURE 2   Spectral loss data for silica fibers.

LASERS

The year 1970 was significant for lightwave communications from two points of view. First, the optical fiber loss dropped below 20 dB/km and, second, Hayashi and Panish achieved the first continuous wave operation of a semiconductor laser at room temperature (Hayashi et al., 1970). These two key breakthroughs heralded the arrival of the age of lightwave communications.

Injection semiconductor lasers were first reported in 1962 (Hall et al., 1962; Holonyak and Bevacqua, 1962; Nathan et al., 1962; Quist et al., 1962). They were homojunction devices whose threshold currents for laser action were so high that a practical lightwave communication that would require continuous wave operation at room temperature could not be envisioned. The following advances, important in the eventual continuous wave operation of semiconductor lasers at room temperatures, occurred in rapid succession: (a) the demonstration of a GaAl-AlGaAs heterostructure growth by Woodall et al. (1967); (b) the demonstration of heterojunction lasers by Hayashi, Panish, and their coworkers (Hayashi et al., 1969; Panish et al., 1969); and (c) the demonstration of double heterostructure for a dual-confinement active region by Alferov and colleagues (Alferov et al., 1969) and by Panish et al. (1970). By 1976 the double heterostructure laser structure of Hayashi and Panish had been developed to a point at which estimated life reached a million hours based on extrapolation from aging tests at elevated temperatures (Hartman et al., 1977). Today, the double heterostructure concept for carrier and photon confinement is used in all practical semiconductor lasers for communications and other applications.

To achieve continuous wave laser action at room temperature, even with the double heterostructure concept, lateral confinement (often called guiding) is necessary for both the injected current and the photons. In the GaAs-GaAlAs laser of the early 1970s, this was achieved by using proton bombardment to define an active stripe of the laser (see Figure 3). The proton bombardment makes the exposed material resistive, so that the injected current is confined to the narrow stripe shielded under the tungsten wire. The optical gain thus produced in the stripe provides gain-induced guiding in the lateral dimension. The first-generation lightwave systems, operating with multimode fibers and at approximately 840 nm, used the stripe geometry lasers.

Early in 1975 it became clear to many people working in the field that the region of low fiber loss was going to shift to longer wavelengths as the concentration of OH impurities in the fibers was being reduced. Further, the zero dispersion wavelength could now match with a low-loss region at 1.3 μm (see Appendix A). The use of zero dispersion necessitated the use of single-

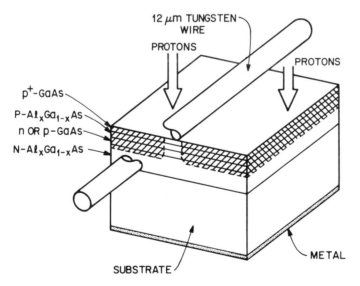

FIGURE 3   Proton-bombarded stripe geometry laser.

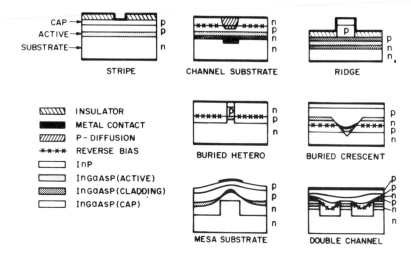

FIGURE 4   Six structures for single transverse-mode lasers.

mode fibers, and the long wavelength required going to ternary and quaternary compounds for lasers. Along with the single-mode fibers came the need for single transverse-mode lasers for efficient coupling of the laser output into the fiber. The six new structures shown in Figure 4 accomplish this to various degrees. The amount of lateral optical guiding determines the size of the mode, that is, mode volume, and therefore determines the "single-modedness" of the laser. Where the optical guiding is provided either by the lateral loss or by lateral mismatch of dielectric constants, they are called strongly guided structures. Guiding achieved only by the lateral definition of the gain (gain guiding) is a weak guiding process. These latter structures are thus called weakly guiding structures.

STATUS OF LASERS FOR COMMUNICATIONS

During the past several years the number of optical fiber communications systems has grown spectacularly. Most have been high-capacity systems in long-distance communications networks Nearly all of the systems installed today use single-mode silica fiber and InGaAsP/InP-based semiconductor lasers operating at a wavelength of 1,300 nm. This section will describe the key parameters of these commercially available lasers and the potential for improved performance as suggested by laboratory results. It will also discuss the principal current areas of laser research to give a sense of the types of communications lasers that might be possible in the future.

A variety of laser structures are used today in communications systems. Some of the most popular are shown in Figure 4. Nearly all are of the general class of buried heterostructures and are produced by various methods of liquid-phase epitaxy (LPE). In some, a planar active layer is grown first and subsequently patterned and covered by an LPE overgrowth to bury the laser stripe—hence the name *buried heterostructure*. In another major design, the active layer is grown in a V-shaped groove to give lateral confinement of carriers and light. These various types are all characterized by a narrow active stripe (1.5–3 μm) and strong index guiding. Despite differences in details of design, the performance of the various types is not very different. The major variables characterizing all communications lasers are optical power output, modulation bandwidth, reliability, frequency spectrum, and cost. The following is a summary of the current status and future prospects in each of these five categories.

Optical Power Output Nearly all lasers available today are capable of generating at least 10 mW of optical power at the facet of the laser chip. Some can be driven as high as 30 mW. Laboratory studies have reported outputs as high as 100 mW (and higher for laser arrays). However, for packaged communications lasers, the output available at the fiber pigtail is typically 1 mW average during modulation (0 dBm). This is lower than the maximum facet power due to a 4- to 5-dB laser-to-fiber coupling loss and the need to operate the laser at less than its maximum power to maintain good reliability. The 0-dBm output is adequate for systems operating up to several hundred megabits per second with less than 30-km repeater spacings, but only marginal for bit rates over 1 Gbit/s at 30 km or for systems (e.g., undersea cables) requiring long repeater spacings.

Modulation Bandwidth Nearly all lasers available today can be modulated at 500 MHz. This is easily adequate for most systems in use. With minor optimization, most laser designs can be stretched to the 1.7-Gbit/s rate that is the fastest system commercially available. Laboratory tests of specially optimized laser designs have been reported in excess of 5 GHz, whereas the world record (obtained at 77 K) is 36 GHz (Bowers, 1985).

Reliability The most reliable lasers are used for undersea applications. Such lasers typically have a mean life in excess of 100,000 hours at room temperature. In terrestrial systems lasers with somewhat shorter lifetimes can often be used and are usually available for a significantly lower cost. Such lifetimes are nevertheless considerably less than those usually specified for most telephone equipment, for which a million hours is a typical desirable mean lifetime. Reliability is a severe problem for lasers that must withstand temperatures up to 70°C. These temperatures typically are used for accelerated aging tests, and lifetimes of 1,000 hours or less are considered good by today's standards. Clearly, there is room for improvement in high-temperature reliability. Such conditions can be met today only with thermoelectric coolers in the laser package.

Frequency Spectrum   Nearly all lasers sold today operate in the fundamental transverse mode but with multiple longitudinal modes. The mean spectral width is typically about 5 nm and consists of several longitudinal modes spaced by roughly 1 nm. For 1,300-nm lasers, such a spectral width is acceptable in most systems because the fiber dispersion crosses zero at this wavelength (Appendix A). However, for 1,550-nm lasers that use the low-loss window in silica fibers, such a multifrequency spectrum is unacceptable for information systems operating faster than several tens of megabits per second because of the significant fiber dispersion at this wavelength.

Therefore, single-frequency lasers have recently been developed that meet system needs at 1,550 nm. A few vendors now offer distributed feedback (DFB) lasers for systems requiring a single-frequency laser (Kogelnik and Shank, 1971). DFB lasers are also useful at 1,300 nm for systems operating above 1 Gbit/s. The linewidth of a single longitudinal mode of a semiconductor is about 100 MHz at 1 mW of continuous wave output. This is determined by the laser cavity length of 300 μm. However, under modulation, the linewidth broadens to roughly 10 GHz because of frequency chirp as the laser current is changed (Olsson et al., 1984). This chirp effect will be a problem for future 1,550-nm long-haul systems operating beyond 1 Gbit/s even with single-frequency lasers.

Cost   Communications lasers currently cost about $1,000 or more, depending on their power, wavelength, bandwidth, spectral purity, and reliability. This cost is acceptable for high-capacity trunk systems but is at least an order of magnitude too high for use in local systems between homes and offices. The price is high because it must cover the sophisticated testing needed to ensure reliability and, to a lesser degree, the cost of the mechanical package. That the AlGaAs lasers for compact audio disc (CD) players now cost roughly $10 gives hope for a

considerable reduction of cost in future InGaAsP communications lasers as well. The extreme cost reduction obtained for CD
lasers has been due largely to a highly uniform materials
technology, modest reliability needs, a simple package, and
limited testing before final assembly. Some, but not all, of these
factors may translate to communications lasers, so that a goal of
lowering costs to $100 might not be unreasonable in the future.

FUTURE TRENDS IN LASERS

The future trends in communications lasers can be described by
a brief summary of the current frontiers of semiconductor laser
research. The major research areas today are materials, frequency control, linewidth, and integration.

Materials   Nearly all InGaAsP lasers sold today are produced
by liquid-phase epitaxy (LPE) (Casey and Panish, 1978). This is
a convenient method for laboratory research and has been
successfully scaled up for production. However, the epitaxial
layers grown in this way are not as uniform as those possible with
newer growth techniques, such as metal-organic chemical vapor
deposition (MOCVD) (Dupuis, 1984) or molecular beam epitaxy
(MBE) (Cho, 1983; Cho and Arthur, 1975). It is generally
believed that MOCVD and MBE offer the potential of higher
manufacturing yield and hence lower costs. Thus, there is
considerable research into these growth methods.

Perhaps the most exotic and promising of the new methods is
gas-source MBE (Panish and Temkin, 1985). This was developed because the conventional MBE technique using solid
elemental sources, such as gallium or arsenic, could not grow
good-quality material that contained both arsenic and phospho-
rus. The fact that gas-source MBE can produce atomically sharp
interfaces between layers of different compositions and hence
band gaps (see Figure 5) gives the potential for a rich array of
novel structures. It is well known that AlGaAs lasers grown by
MBE using tailored band gaps and multi-quantum wells
(MQWs) give superior performance (Tsang, 1981); hence, it is
expected that such techniques will also be beneficial when
applied to InGaAsP lasers.

New materials are important for semiconductor lasers operating at wavelengths beyond 1,550 nm. Fiber research is currently focusing on new materials in the search for ultralow-loss
fiber in the wavelength range between 2 and 5 μm (see Appendix A). Lasers are being studied in this region as well. In general,
the materials systems being studied are based on either GaSb or

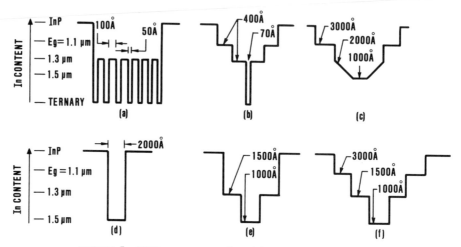

FIGURE 5   Different types of multi-quantum well laser structures fabricated using molecular beam epitaxy.

InAs, since InP-based materials cannot operate beyond about 1,650 nm. The best result to date for room-temperature operation of a continuous wave laser is slightly beyond 2 μm using LPE growth in a GaSb-based system (Caneau et al., 1985). Considerable effort in the 3- to 4-μm range in InAs-based systems has produced lasers at 77 K, but none at room temperature. This trend toward poorer temperature performance with longer wavelengths is expected theoretically; it may ultimately limit the commercial appeal of this wavelength range for all but special situations in which cryogenic laser packages are acceptable.

Frequency Control   The recent trend toward single-frequency lasers, such as DFB and cleaved-coupled-cavity (C^3) lasers (Tsang et al., 1983), is the best example of this sort of research. In recent DFB laser research, unwanted longitudinal modes have been suppressed more than 40,000 to 1 relative to the main mode (Tsang et al., 1985). Gratings for DFB lasers are typically fabricated by holographic photolithography. However, recent results (Temkin et al., 1985) with electron beam lithography promise even higher resolution and greater control over the detailed shape of the grating (see Figure 6). In spite of the recent progress with single-frequency lasers, much still remains to be done. In particular, even though the longitudinal mode control is excellent, the fabrication process cannot yet be sufficiently controlled to set absolute frequency standards, or channels, with a precision and reproducibility anywhere near the linewidth of the laser.

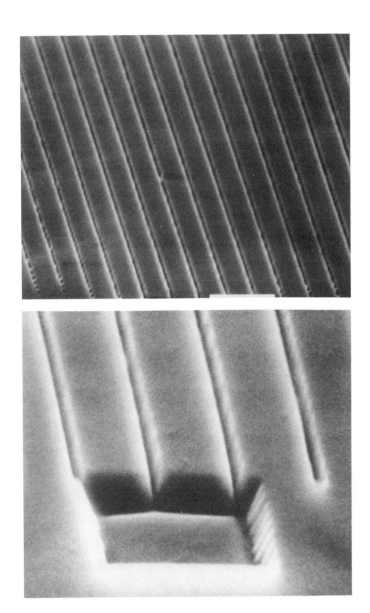

FIGURE 6   Distributed feedback grating.

Linewidth   Although the single-longitudinal-mode, 1.5-μm lasers have dramatically improved the performance of fiber-optic communication systems, they are not without problems. Under continuous wave operation, a typical DFB (300 μm long) or C^3 laser has a linewidth of about 100 MHz. Under direct amplitude modulation, however, the linewidth is broadened, or chirped,

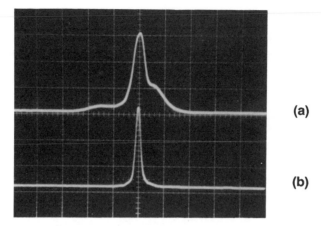

(a)

(b)

FIGURE 7   Chirp-induced broadening of laser linewidth (1-Å/div horizontal scale): with modulation (a); without modulation (b).

as a result of the carrier density dynamics during modulation of the laser (Olsson et al., 1984). Typically, this chirp gives a modulated linewidth of approximately 10 GHz (1 Å), as shown in Figure 7. For data rates below 1 Gbit/s, the chirping is of little consequence to communication systems. For the very high bit-rate systems, however, the wavelength chirping of the lasers, coupled with the dispersion of the fiber, can give a substantial penalty. For example, in the terabit-km/s experiment described later in this paper, the 10 channels incurred chirp penalties between 1 and 3.5 dB. That is, the receiver needed between 25 and 225 percent more power to achieve a given error rate than would have been required if the laser did not chirp. Two methods have been demonstrated to solve the chirp problem: injection locking and external modulation (Olsson et al., 1985). Injection locking has been used in a 2-Gbit/s system, and external modulation has been used in a 4-Gbit/s experiment. Both experiments demonstrated the elimination of any chirp-related penalties. With these techniques, injection locking and external modulation, the optical communication systems have become so sophisticated that, for the first time, the linewidth of the transmitted signal is given by the information bandwidth. The coding of the information, however, is still the most primitive (and simplest) possible; only the energy in the transmitted pulses is detected.

The next step in refinement would be a system in which the phase, frequency, and polarization of the optical wave are significant. This leads us to coherent optical communication

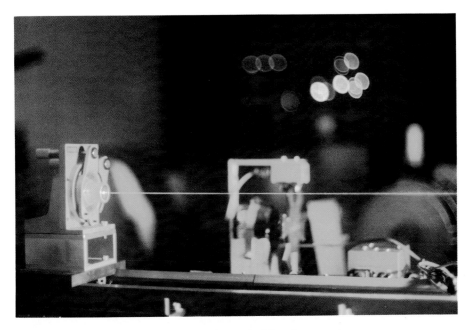

PLATE 1   The highly collimated laser beam inside a laser cavity.

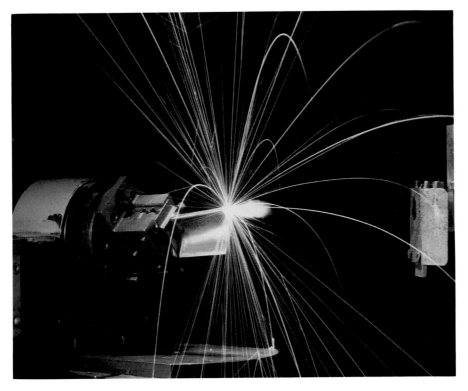

PLATE 2   Drilling holes in a turbine blade with a pulsed laser beam.

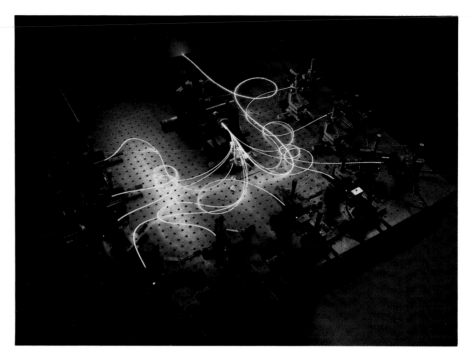

PLATE 3   Wavelength division multiplexer system.

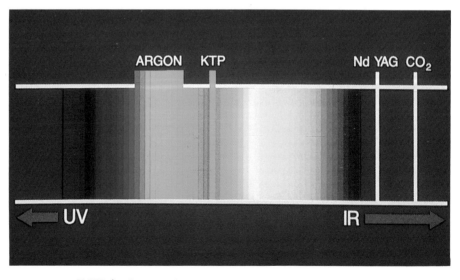

PLATE 4   Commonly used lasers in clinical medicine.

systems that put even greater demands on the lasers. For successful operation of a coherent optical communication system, the phase noise of the lasers must be minimal. This severely restricts the linewidth of both the transmitter and the local oscillator laser. In direct detection systems, the chirp penalty is eliminated for laser linewidths equal to or less than the information bandwidth. Coherent systems, in contrast, require linewidths that are only 1/30 to 1/1,000 of the information bandwidth. Phase-shift keyed homodyne systems require the narrowest linewidth, and amplitude-shift keyed heterodyne systems are the most linewidth tolerant. DFB and C^3 lasers, although operating in a single longitudinal mode, do not have sufficiently narrow linewidths or good frequency stability for coherent applications. By operating the semiconductor laser in an external cavity, the Q, or "quality factor," of the longitudinal modes is increased, and the linewidth of the laser is dramatically decreased. Figure 8 shows the beat spectrum of two 1.5-μm external cavity lasers. The width of the beat spectrum 60 dB down from the peak is 4 MHz, which indicates full width at half-maximum (FWHM) spectral width of 2 kHz for each laser (Olsson and van der Ziel, 1987).

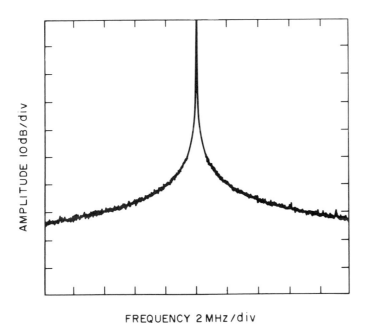

FIGURE 8   Beat spectrum of two 1.5-μm external cavity lasers.

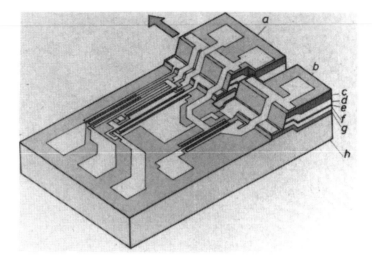

FIGURE 9   Optical electronic integrated circuit. (a) Laser; (b) photodetector; (c) GaAs; (d) GaAlAs; (e) GaAlAs (active layer); (f) GaAlAs; (g) GaAs (conducting layer); and (h) semi-insulating GaAs.

Integration   Many investigators believe that the ultimate scheme to reduce cost and improve performance is opto-electronic integrated circuits (OEICs) (Matsueda et al., 1984). Considerable work is being done on this subject in Japan. Figure 9 shows an example of an optical electronic circuit of this type—a laser monolithically integrated with a small amplifier circuit. Such OEICs range from simple laser arrays to proposals for integrated regenerators and complete integrated optical electronic wideband switching modules. Such complex circuits will probably not be actually used for some time, but the potential for significant cost reduction in high-volume products is a major force behind such work.

DETECTORS

In the last few years, along with the parallel efforts in reducing the optical fiber losses and improving semiconductor laser performance, there has been an intense research and development effort on photodetectors for optical communications. Several important technological and material developments have driven and motivated this effort: (1) the development of low-loss, low-dispersion fibers at 1.3- to 1.55-μm wavelengths; (2) the availability of high-quality and low-doped epitaxial alloys (InGaAsP) and InP grown by liquid-phase and vapor-phase epitaxy (Stillman et al., 1983); and (3) the impressive advances in heterojunction research. These advances include the growth of high-quality heterojunctions and superlattices by MBE (Cho, 1983; Cho and Arthur, 1975) and MOCVD (Dupuis, 1984); better experimental (Margaritondo, 1986) and theoretical (Harrison, 1985) understanding of band discontinuities and perpendicular transport in heterostructures (Capasso et al., 1986); and the realization of the enormous degrees of freedom afforded by heterojunction and superlattices in device design (band-gap engineering) (Capasso, 1985). The detectors used in optical communications are PIN photodiodes, avalanche detectors, and photoconductors (see Appendix B).

STATUS OF LIGHTWAVE COMMUNICATIONS

The light sources used in today's optical communication systems, regardless of type, differ little in wavelength, output power, modulation bandwidth, or electrical power requirements. These quantities vary at most by 2 orders of magnitude between the different types of light sources. However, a variation of 10 orders of magnitude is seen in the emission linewidth of the light sources. A typical light-emitting diode (LED) has an emission linewidth of 1,000 Å (2×10^{13} Hz) at a 1.3-μm wavelength. A 1.5-μm external cavity semiconductor laser, on the other hand, has a linewidth of a few kilohertz (Olsson and van der Ziel, 1987). Table 1 lists the most commonly used light sources and their respective linewidths. Not surprisingly, this large variation in emission linewidth has a profound effect on the performance of optical communication systems. In effect, the evolution of the optical communication technology has been the record of a quest to reduce and control the linewidth of the light source. One example of this is a 20-Mbit/s data rate system using an LED with a linewidth of 1,000 Å. In this case, the linewidth is a million times larger than the information bandwidth, hardly an efficient ap-

TABLE 1   Linewidths of Important Light Sources Used in Lightwave Communications

Device	Linewidth (Hz)
Light-emitting diode	10^{13}
Multimode laser	10^{12}
Single-mode laser	10^{8}
External cavity laser	10^{3}

proach and not much different from Hertz's first radio transmission experiments using an open-air spark as the transmitter.

The following section describes the first lightwave communication system to reach an information-carrying capacity of more than 1 terabit-km/s. This is followed by a discussion of the system limitations imposed by the linewidth of the light sources listed in Table 1 and by examples of current state-of-the-art performance. See Appendix C for a description of a coherent lightwave communication system approaching the theoretical limit of performance.

TERABIT-KM/S EXPERIMENT

In this system demonstration (Hegarty et al., 1985) of close-spaced wavelength division multiplexing with ultrahigh capacity, 10 single-frequency DFB lasers were multiplexed into a single 68-km transmission fiber. The experimental details are shown in Figure 10.

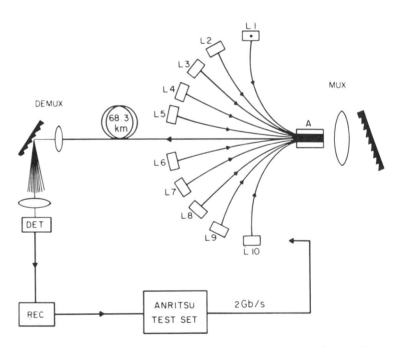

FIGURE 10   Setup for a 10-laser wavelength division multiplex lightwave system.

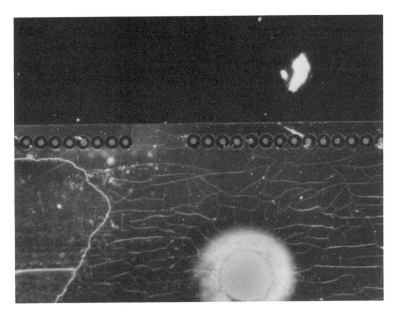

FIGURE 11   Wavelength division multiplexer.

The lasers employed in this experiment were heteroepitaxially ridge overgrown (HRO) DFB lasers (Tsang et al., 1985). The pure single-mode operation of these lasers, even under high-speed modulation, was essential for achieving the narrow channel spacing, low cross talk, and error-free operation of the system. The lasers used a second-order grating, and the mode rejection ratio—the ratio of the dominant mode power to the power in the next largest mode—was between 400:1 and 10,000:1 at a 2-Gbit/s modulation. The laser wavelengths were between 1.53 and 1.56 μm.

The multiplexer (Figure 11) had 22 channels, consisting of 23 single-mode fibers brought together in a linear array. The core-to-core spacing in the array was 24 μm, and the free ends of the 22 input fibers were pigtailed with microlenses for coupling to the lasers (Plate 3). The remaining fiber was the output channel, and its free end was spliced to the transmission fiber. Coupling between the input fibers and the output fiber was achieved with a 2.5-cm lens and a 600 1/mm grating. The resulting channel spacing was 13.5 Å, and the average coupling loss between the input and output fiber was 3 dB. Demultiplexing at the end of the 68-km transmission fiber was achieved with a grating and with the receiver photodetector acting as the spatial filter. The overall cross talk between adjacent channels

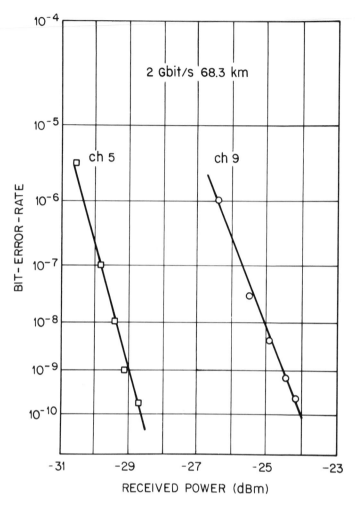

FIGURE 12 Received bit error rates for channels 5 and 9 of the wavelength division multiplex system.

was less than −23 dB, with most of the cross talk originating in the demultiplexer.

The almost pure silica-core transmission fiber had an average loss (including splice losses) of 0.22 dB/km for the 10 lasers, and the dispersion at 1.55 μm was 19 ps/km nm. The receiver used an avalanche photodetector, and the receiver sensitivity at 2 Gbit/s was −32 dBm. The system performance was evaluated with all 10 lasers providing full power into the fiber and by sequentially applying a 2-Gbit/s pseudorandom nonreturn to zero modulation to each laser. The received bit pattern was compared with the transmitted pattern, and the bit error rate (BER) was recorded as a function of received power. For all channels, a BER of less than 1×10^{-9} was achieved, and the BER was independent of the presence of the other channels. BER curves, a recording of the system error rate versus the received power, for the channels requiring the least (channel 5) and the most (channel 9) power for obtaining a 10^9 BER is shown in Figure 12. The difference between the two channels is mainly due to the laser chirping effect. To measure the cross talk, the laser corresponding to the selected channel was turned off, and the photocurrent resulting from all the other nine channels was measured. The ratio of this photocurrent to the signal photocurrent, when the laser for this channel was operated, was less than -23 dB (0.5 percent). This level of cross talk is negligible as confirmed with the BER measurements. This system demonstration is significant in several respects. It is the first optical communication system that is even attempting to get close to the possible capacity of fiber-optic systems. This system uses a third of the bandwidth of the best LED system but has more than 200 times the capacity. It is also the first demonstration of close-spaced wavelength division multiplexing, a necessary technique if the ultimate capacity of the fiber is going to be reached. The demonstrated capacity corresponds to 21 million voice channels-kilometers. When buying a 300-page book for $10, the price is approximately 1.5×10^{-6} per bit of information. At this price per bit, 20 Gbit/s for 1 year corresponds to $1 trillion.

The first optical communication systems to be developed, LED-based systems using multimode fiber, are in general limited by the modal dispersion of the fiber. A typical system is the SLIC-96 loop feeder operating at a data rate of 90 Mbit/s and a repeater spacing of 20 km. The problem of modal dispersion was solved by introducing single-mode fiber. Because of the large spot size of regular surface-emitting LEDs, only a small fraction of the light can be coupled into the fiber. This, plus the increased output power and modulation bandwidth available from lasers, spurred the development of 1.3-μm wavelength lasers. However, with special edge-emitting LEDs with small spot size, as much as 30 μW of power has been coupled into a single-mode fiber, and a transmission distance of 35 km at 180 Mbit/s has been demonstrated. Conventional semiconductor lasers emit light in a few (3–10) longitudinal modes spaced about

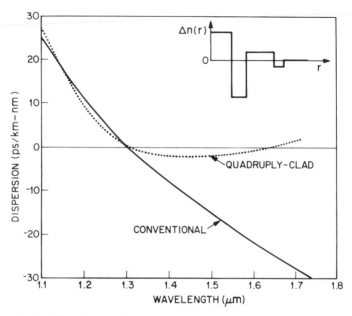

FIGURE 13 Chromatic dispersion in single-mode silica fibers as a function of wavelength. The solid line is for conventional step index fiber. Note the zero dispersion region near 1.3 μm, which permits the use of multimode laser sources without sacrificing bit rate or distance between repeaters. The dotted curve is the measured dispersion of an experimental quadruply clad fiber, with an index profile shown in the inset.

10 Å apart. The linewidth of a laser with five modes is 10^{12} Hz at 1.3 μm, which is the first loss minimum of silica optical fibers, as seen in Figure 2. Fortunately, at a 1.3-μm wavelength, the chromatic and waveguide dispersion in the fiber cancels (Figure 13). While the broad linewidth of the source is a terrible waste of available bandwidth, the large linewidth does not impose a dispersion penalty at 1.3 μm, and the transmission systems are loss limited. For example, the transatlantic undersea cable TAT-8 (see Figure 14) uses 1.3-μm lasers at a data rate of 296 Mbit/s and a repeater spacing of about 50 km.

At 1.5 μm, the transmission loss of the optical fiber is only about half of that at 1.3 μm; therefore, in principle, the repeater spacing can be doubled by switching to a 1.5-μm light source in the transmitter. The dispersion, however, which was minimal at 1.3 μm, is substantial—typically, 18 ps/km nm—at a 1.5-μm wavelength. The hard-sought breakthrough was the achievement of single-longitudinal-mode operation of 1.5-μm wavelength lasers. Some conventional semiconductor lasers emit predominantly in a single longitudinal mode. Under continuous wave operation, as much as 99 percent of the output power may be concentrated in one mode. Continuous wave measurements, however, are poor indicators of how the laser will perform in a communication system. The requirement for optical communication systems is that the laser emits in one longitudinal mode all the time and under amplitude modulation. No conventional Fabry-Perot semiconductor laser fulfills this requirement. As described above, the two most successful laser structures for achieving dynamic single-mode operation are the distributed feedback (DFB) (Kogelnik and Shank, 1971) and cleaved-coupled-cavity (C^3) (Tsang et al., 1983) lasers. With the advent of these narrow linewidth lasers, the improvement in capacity, transmission distance, and bit rate of fiber communication systems was dramatic. System experiments over 103 km at 420 Mbit/s, 130 km at 2 Gbit/s, and 117 km at 4 Gbit/s were demonstrated in rapid succession. Further, the use of single-longitudinal-mode lasers opens up the possibility of close-spaced wavelength division multiplexing (WDM) and thereby makes possible more efficient use of the available fiber bandwidth. The state of the art in WDM is represented by the recent 10-channel,

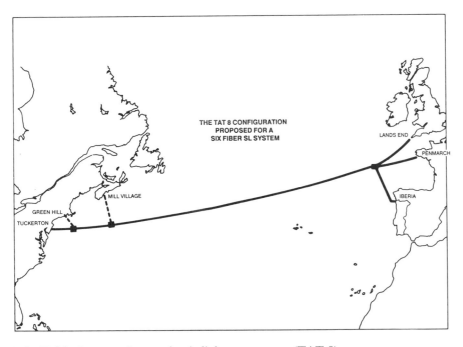

FIGURE 14   Layout of transatlantic lightwave system (TAT-8).

20-Gbit/s, 68-km transmission experiment with the highest capacity of any optical communication system, 1.37 terabit-km/s (see the box on p. 60).

OPTICAL PROCESSING

The possibility of optical information processing is tantalizing for several reasons. All-optical systems would have multiple intrinsic advantages over electronic systems in speed, parallelism, and low cross talk. In addition, light propagates in free space with negligible dispersion and loss; light beams can intersect in space without cross talk; and a number of beams can be simultaneously operated on by one element, then separated. However, several difficult problems must be solved to use these advantages. In particular, methods of switching, storage, regeneration, and performing logic operations with light have to be devised in analogy with their electronic counterparts. These functions are routinely obtained with electronics today. However, it is clear that the optical versions of these and related operations are now in their infancy. The requirements for such a computer or information processor have yet to be clearly defined, and in particular, it is not clear what architecture would be suitable for these kinds of problems: either a limited number of devices operating at extremely high speeds or a massive parallel network of devices operating at lower speeds. The particular characteristics of the optical devices will help to determine a suitable architecture. In fact, even if suitable devices existed today for high-speed optical processing in parallel architectures, algorithms for programming and operating massively parallel machines have yet to be devised.

Although it may not be necessary to use lasers for optical information processing and computing, laser light has several advantages over conventional light sources, some of which can and have been exploited to make new devices and components. In particular, the highly focusable intensity that is obtainable with lasers makes nonlinear optics possible for use in optical logic and switching applications, and the generation of picosecond optical pulses with mode-locked semiconductor lasers makes high bit rates feasible in optical systems.

OPTICAL SWITCHING

Optical switching serves the function of routing a signal into various alternative paths. Several methods have been devised for

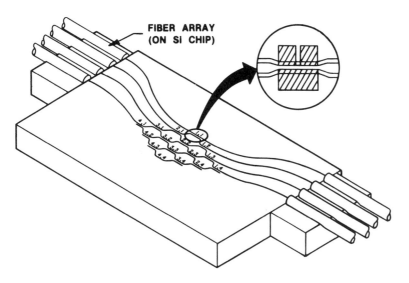

FIGURE 15   Schematic representation of a 4 × 4 Ti:LiNbO$_3$ directional coupler switch array.

such switching of light, notably acousto-optic and electro-optic beam deflectors. One necessary component of an optical processor or computer is a device that can interchange the connections in order to reroute the paths of the individual output beams into other inputs. In principle, a switching device should be capable of interconnecting any output channel to any input channel with low cross talk and completely within a single machine cycle. At this time, we do not know what kind of cycle times might be used or what data rates in each channel might be necessary. Optical crossbars have been constructed using electro-optical materials such as lithium niobate in waveguide structures (Schmidt and Kaminow, 1974; Schmidt and Kogelnik, 1976; Alferness, 1981). Details of a 4 × 4 switch (see Figures 15 and 16) have already been published (McCaughan and Bogert, 1985). Recently, as

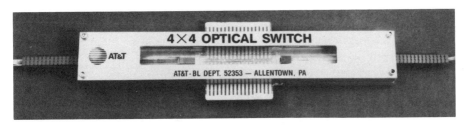

FIGURE 16   Packaged and pigtailed 4 × 4 optical switch.

many as eight channels have been switched at rates of several hundred megahertz with cross talk levels of -30 dB per channel (Granesrand et al., 1986). For optical processing applications as many as 10,000 switching elements are envisioned. This seems well beyond the range of existing fabrication technology.

OPTICAL MODULATION

Electro-optic modulation (Reinhart and Miller, 1972) and optical switching (Shelton et al., 1978) have been demonstrated in GaAs/GaAlAs heterostructure waveguides. This low-loss waveguide geometry creates a close coupling between the applied modulating (or switching) field and the propagating optical field, thus allowing for efficient modulation (or switching) by means of the linear electro-optic effect. Several types of modulators, including electroabsorption, phase, and polarization modulators, have shown good performance. For example, a polarization modulator has been fabricated that requires less than 10 V to produce an extinction ratio of 20 dB. One advantage of these semiconductor devices is the possibility of integrating them with lasers, detectors, and transistors to create integrated optical circuits (see Figure 9). Efficient optical modulation can also be obtained at room temperature with excitonic electroabsorptive effects in quantum well devices (Miller et al., 1985a). By integrating single quantum wells into waveguide structures, modulations as large as 10 dB have been obtained with logic-level drive voltages (Wiener et al., 1985), and switching times of 100 ps have been demonstrated (Wood et al., 1985). The intrinsic response time of the excitonic electroabsorption has been found (Knox et al., 1986) to be at least as short as 330 fs. The use of quantum well modulators at the board-and-chip level is considered feasible, since the dimensions, electrical drive requirements and operating temperatures, and wavelengths are consistent with those of existing and experimental high-speed GaAs logic chips.

OPTICAL STORAGE

An optical computer will need an optical memory, with optical inputs and outputs. The present generation of optical storage discs uses electronic drivers and readout devices, and therefore is not included in this discussion. Optical fibers have been suggested as a means of storing optical information. However, the speed of light and the rate at which photons are lost to dissipative processes would seem to militate against the storage of optical information in fibers except for short times. To store information for only 1 μs, a fiber 300 m long is required. In certain types of optical computers, there will nevertheless probably be a need for relatively short-term memories, but with high capacity and rapid access. To store information for longer periods, longer fibers are required; however, signal losses eventually dominate the storage time. A method to counteract the loss is required.

Many kilometers of single-mode optical fiber can be coiled onto small spools a few centimeters in diameter without severe loss due to bending (J. W. Simpson, personal communication). With ends coupled together to form a reentrant loop, and with Raman amplification used to compensate for recirculating signal losses, a large amount of information can be stored for a surprisingly long time (Mollenauer et al., 1985). For example, a loop 40 km long would have an access time of about 200 ms, and assuming a 100-ps spacing between adjacent pulses, its capacity would be about 2 Mbits. Furthermore, with wavelength multiplexing, this capacity could be increased by 10 times or more. Storage times of tens of milliseconds should be possible, limited by noise effects. Erasure is provided by temporarily turning off the optical pump power and allowing the signal to dissipate naturally.

Another promising technique of optical data storage is that of spectral hole burning (Gutierrez et al., 1982). By using a relatively intense monochromatic pump laser to induce a photochemical reaction, a spectrally narrow homogeneously broadened "hole" (i.e., frequency gap) can be written in an inhomogeneously broadened optical transition. This information can then be read by using a weak optical probe beam. This approach offers the possibility of greatly increasing the storage density by the ratio of the inhomogeneous to homogeneous linewidths, which is typically approximately 10^3. Since the conventional planar geometry optical memories (for example, the optical discs) are limited by diffraction to a maximum of 10^8 bits/cm^2 (corresponding to 1 bit per square wavelength), the spectral hole burning technique can increase the density to 10^{11} bits/cm^2. The information can be stored for hours at 4 K, since the optical saturation is based on photochemical processes that have negligible thermal reversibility at low temperature. At present, up to 30 bits of information have been written in a doped polymer film (see Figure 17) with spectral holes as narrow as 100 MHz. Research aimed at making this a practical technology is directed toward increasing the sensitivity of the recording medium by several orders of magnitude to allow nanosecond read/write times.

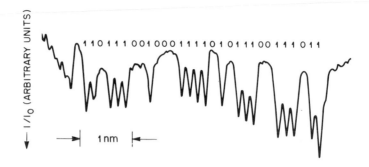

WAVELENGTH

FIGURE 17   Sequence of 30 bits written onto a doped polymer film at 4 K. The presence or absence of spectral holes is designated by ones and zeros, respectively (Gutierrez et al., 1982).

OPTICAL LOGIC AND BISTABILITY

The ability to perform logic functions using optical inputs and outputs must be considered a basic requirement of an optical computer or information processor. Of course, it would be possible to build hybrid devices wherein optical inputs are detected and fed into the inputs of conventional electronic logic elements, and the output signal is then converted to an optical signal by an LED or laser diode. The losses due to inefficiency at every conversion stage cannot be tolerated if we are to construct a system of high-density, fast-switching devices operating at high data rates. If light itself could be used to control other light beams through optical logic devices, a significant simplification would be possible. Interactions with light are generally weaker than is desirable; therefore, considerable effort is required to produce optical logic devices at present.

Bistability, which is essential to optical logic, has been shown in a variety of optical devices. In particular, bistability as a result of absorption and dispersion changes, electroabsorption (self-electro-optic effect devices [SEED]), and index variations (optical logic etalons) have been shown. The availability of optically bistable devices of high speed, low dissipation, good stability, and small size will make it possible to implement true optical logic devices such as gates, inverters, and saturable amplifiers in large arrays that can be combined to perform optical processing and computation functions. At present, no specific devices satisfying these requirements have been implemented.

The first optical bistable devices used nonlinear Fabry-Perot cavities and optical beams of sufficient intensity to change the characteristic of the medium within the cavity to perform the desired optical logic (Szoke et al., 1969; Seidel, 1971; Gibbs et al., 1976, 1978). Bistability has been demonstrated in several experiments. In particular, such devices constructed with MBE-grown GaAs/GaAlAs superlattice structure (Gibbs et al., 1982) (see Figure 18) or other semiconductors have a number of advantages, including a fast operating speed (10-ns switching times) and operating at a wavelength near 0.9 μm and at room temperature (see Figure 19 for input/output characteristics of such a device). So far, the power requirements are large—about 10 nJ for a 100-μm^2 device. Such bistable devices are suitable for continuous wave processing and memory applications.

SEED uses the electroabsorption in a GaAs MQW in combination with a feedback loop to produce bistability with a single input wavelength (Miller et al., 1985b) (see Figure 20). A bias field is applied with a constant current source perpendicular to the plane of the quantum well, which shifts the excitonic resonance. When light is incident on the device, the induced photocurrent reduces the voltage across the quantum well, which shifts the resonance back in the direction of the unbiased excitonic absorption. This in turn reduces the absorption, which increases the intensity, and the device becomes optically bistable. Switching speed is limited by the RC time constant of the device, and speeds of nanoseconds to seconds have been demonstrated. Large transmission modulation (>10 dB) can be obtained with these devices.

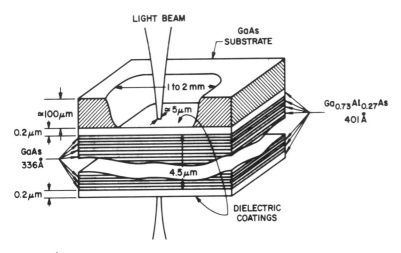

FIGURE 18   GaAs-GaAlAs superlattice structure used for room temperature optical bistability.

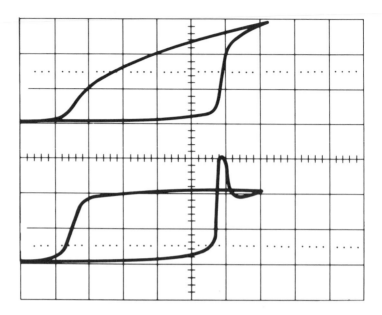

FIGURE 19   Output versus input characteristics for the device shown in Figure 18. Upper trace shows the entire output. Lower trace shows output corresponding to the central part of the beam.

Optical logic etalons (OLE) are nonlinear Fabry-Perot devices (Jewell et al., 1986; Lee et al., 1986) (see Figure 21), similar in construction to the bistable devices discussed above. OLE devices, however, need not be bistable. An intense pump beam induces a change in the index of refraction of the nonlinear material in the etalon and shifts the resonance of the etalon, causing a change in the transmission of a probe beam. Cycle times of 30 ps have been obtained with 20-pJ input energy. Further, a 2 × 2 array of NOR gates (see Figure 22) has been operated at 82 MHz. The OLE is a three-port, all-optical gate that operates with two different wavelengths and is complementary to other approaches. In normal operation, the control beam wavelength is shorter than the probe beam wavelength in order to provide the third port. Were such devices the only ones available for optical logic, the total number of sequential logic operations would be limited, because the probe wavelength would continue to shift down monotonically in each operation. Recently, complementary OLE devices have been demonstrated (J. L. Jewell, personal communication) for which the control beam has a wavelength longer than that of the probe beam. Cascading now need not cause a monotonic shift in the operat-

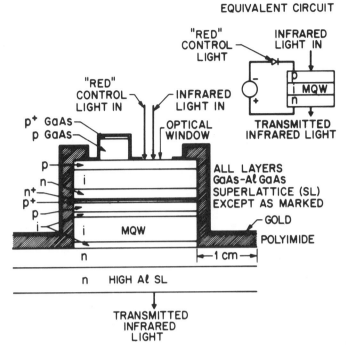

FIGURE 20   Details of construction of a self-electro-optic effect device.

ing wavelength. Operation near a 1.55-μm wavelength has been recently demonstrated (K. Tai, personal communication).

An important requirement of optical logic devices is that they be cascadable, or that the output of one device can drive the input of at least the next device, if not several inputs. In optical terms, this means that there must be enough optical gain in the system to offset losses. This is not easily obtained in large arrays. However, various approaches have been suggested. One that is particularly interesting is the use of optically bistable elements

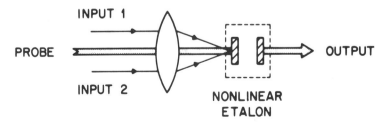

FIGURE 21   Schematic of an optical logic etalon.

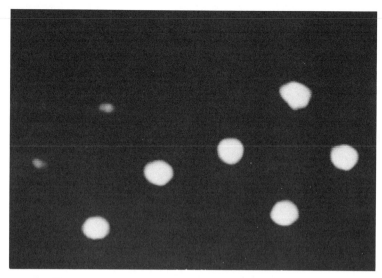

FIGURE 22   A 2 × 2 array of optical logic etalons. Left frame: two devices turned on. Right frame: all four devices turned on. (SOURCE: Jewell et al., 1986).

that are biased near their switching transition by a strong beam. A weak signal beam falls on the elements and switches the devices into high output mode, thus providing net differential gain. This scheme removes the coherence between the signal and amplified signal beams, but provides the desirable modal isolation and saturable output characteristics for regenerative systems. Again, however, the problems of scaling too many elements for massively parallel systems operating at high data rates are formidable.

DIRECTIONS IN OPTICAL PROCESSING

In conclusion, the requirements for optical processing and computing are not yet clearly defined. Some of the basic elements that will be required for a full-scale operational processor have, in fact, been demonstrated in a limited way, that is, single devices at moderate performance levels; however, no existing technology seems directly scalable to the large number of elements and high operating speeds that would allow us to take full advantage of the properties of light. The physical processes that have been exploited to date are either too slow or not efficient enough to allow close packing and high-speed operation. In fact, most technologies are so far from meeting the requirements envisioned at this time that a breakthrough is probably needed.

CONCLUSION

Lightwave communications, optical switching, and computation are only three areas of the many in which lasers are playing a pivotal role. But even in these areas, we can see that lasers, together with a number of significant achievements in related fields, have caused a revolution in communications. In information processing, the impact of laser technology is not yet visible, but if the past is any guide, information processing also will see its capabilities significantly enhanced through a variety of laser applications, many of which are still in the conceptual stage.

ACKNOWLEDGMENTS

I would like to thank Drs. N. A. Olsson, D. V. Lang, E. Capasso, S. L. McCall, and D. S. Chemla for assistance in putting this manuscript together, and Dr. A. M. Glass for critical comments.

REFERENCES

Alferness, R. C. 1981. IEEE J. Quantum Electron. QE-17:946–959.

Alferov, Zh. I., V. M. Andreev, V. I. Korol'kov, E. L. Portnoi, and D. N. Tretyakov. 1969. Sov. Phys. Semicond. 2:843. [Translated from Fiz. Tekh. Poluprovodn. 2:1016 (1968).]

Bowers, J. E. 1985. Electron. Lett. 21:1195.

Caneau, C., A. K. Srivastava, A. G. Dentai, J. L. Zyskind, and M. A. Pollack. 1985. Electron. Lett. 21:815.

Capasso, F. 1985. Physica 129B:92.

Capasso, F., K. Mohammed, and A. Y. Cho. 1986. IEEE J. Quantum Electron. QE-22(September):1853.

Casey, H. C., Jr., and M. B. Panish. 1978. Heterostructure Lasers, Parts A and B. New York: Academic Press.

Cho, A. Y. 1983. Thin Solid Films 100:291.

Cho, A. Y., and J. R. Arthur. 1975. Prog. Solid-State Chem. 10:157.

Dupuis, R. D. 1984. Science 226:623.

Gibbs, H. M., S. L. McCall, and T. N. C. Venkatesan. 1976. Phys. Rev. Lett. 36:1135.

Gibbs, H. M., S. L. McCall, and T. N. C. Venkatesan. 1978. U.S. Patent 4,071,831.

Gibbs, H. M., S. L. McCall, J. L. Jewell, D. A. Weinberger, K. Tai, A. C. Gossard, A. Passner, and W. Wiegmann. 1982. Appl. Phys. Lett. 41:221.

Granesrand, P., L. Thylen, B. Stoltz, K. Bergvall, W. Doldissen, H. Heidrich, and D. Hoffmann. 1986. Integrated and Guided Wave Optics Conference, Atlanta, Ga., February 26–28, Paper WAA-3.

Gutierrez, A. R., J. Friedrich, D. Haarer, and H. Wolfrum. 1982. IBM J. Res. Dev. 26:198–208.

Hall, R. N., G. E. Fenner, J. D. Kingsley, T. J. Foltys, and R. O. Carlson. 1962. Phys. Rev. Lett. 9:366–368.

Harrison, W. A. 1985. J. Vacuum Sci. Technol. B3:1231.

Hartman, R. L., N. E. Schumaker, and R. W. Dixon. 1977. Appl. Phys. Lett. 31:756.

Hayashi, I., M. B. Panish, and P. W. Foy. 1969. IEEE J. Quantum Electron. QE-5:211.

Hayashi, I., M. B. Panish, P. W. Foy, and S. Sumski. 1970. Appl. Phys. Lett. 17:109.

Hegarty, J., N. A. Olsson, and L. Goldner. 1985. Electron. Lett. 21:290–292.

Holonyak, N., Jr., and S. F. Bevacqua. 1962. Appl. Phys. Lett. 1:82–83.

Jewell, J. L., Y. H. Lee, J. F. Duffy, A. C. Gossard, W. Wiegmann, and J. H. English. 1986. P. 32 in Optical Bistability III, Springer Proceedings in Physics, Vol. 8. New York: Springer-Verlag.

Kao, K. C., and G. A. Hochkam. 1966. Proc. IEE 113:1151–1158.

Knox, W. H., D. A. B. Miller, T. C. Damen, D. S. Chemla, C. V. Shank, and A. C. Gossard. 1986. Appl. Phys. Lett. 48:864.

Kogelnik, H., and C. V. Shank. 1971. Appl. Phys. Lett. 18:152.

Lee, Y. H., H. M. Gibbs, J. L. Jewell, J. F. Duffy, T. N. C. Venkatesan, A. C. Gossard, W. Wiegmann, and J. H. English. 1986. Appl. Phys. Lett. 49:486–488.

Margaritondo, G. 1986. Solid-State Electron. 29:123.

Matsueda, H., T. P. Tanaka, and H. Nakano. 1984. Proc. IEE 131(5):299–303.

Mayo, J. S. 1985. The evolution of information technologies. Pp. 7–34 in Information Technologies and Social Transformation, B. R. Guile, ed. Washington, D.C.: National Academy Press.

McCaughan, L., and G. A. Bogert. 1985. Appl. Phys. Lett. 47:348–350.

Miller, D. A. B., D. S. Chemla, T. C. Damen, A. C. Gossard, W. Wiegmann, T. H. Wood, and C. A. Burrus. 1985a. Phys. Rev. B32:1043.

Miller, D. A. B., D. S. Chemla, T. C. Damen, T. H. Wood, C. A. Burrus, A. C. Gossard, and W. Wiegmann. 1985b. IEEE J. Quantum Electron. QE-21:1462.

Mollenauer, L. F., R. H. Stolen, and M. N. Islam. 1985. Opt. Lett. 10:229.

Nathan, M. I., W. P. Dumke, G. Burns, F. H. Dill, Jr., and G. Lasher. 1962. Appl. Phys. Lett. 1:62–64.

Nelson, K. C., D. L. Brownlow, L. G. Cohen, F. D. DiMarcello, R. G. Huff, J. T. Krause, P. J. Lemaire, W. A. Reed, D. S. Shenk, E. A. Sigety, J. R. Simpson, A. Tomita, and K. L. Walker. 1985. J. Lightwave Technol. LT-3(5):935–941.

Olsson, N. A. 1985. Electron. Lett. 21:1085–1087.

Olsson, N. A., and J. P. van der Ziel. 1987. J. Lightwave Technol. (Special Issue on Coherent Communications) LT-5:509–515.

Olsson, N. A., N. K. Dutta, and K.-Y. Liou. 1984. Electron. Lett. 20:121.

Olsson, N. A., H. Temkin, R. A. Logan, L. F. Johnson, G. J. Dolan, J. P. van der Ziel, and J. C. Campbell. 1985. J. Lightwave Technol. LT-3:63–67.

Panish, M. B., and H. Temkin. 1985. J. Vacuum Sci. Technol. B3:657.

Panish, M. B., I. Hayashi, and S. Sumski. 1969. IEEE J. Quantum Electron. QE-5:210.

Panish, M. B., I. Hayashi, and S. Sumski. 1970. Appl. Phys. Lett. 16:326.

Quist, T. M., R. H. Rediker, R. J. Keyes, W. E. Krag, B. Lax, A. L. McWhorter, and H. J. Zeiger. 1962. Appl. Phys. Lett. 1:91–92.

Reinhart, F. K., and B. I. Miller. 1972. Appl. Phys. Lett. 20:36–38.

Schawlow, A. L., and C. H. Townes. 1958. Phys. Rev. 112:1940.

Schmidt, R. V., and I. P. Kaminow. 1974. Appl. Phys. Lett. 25:458–460.

Schmidt, R. V., and H. Kogelnik. 1976. Appl. Phys. Lett. 29:503–505.

Seidel, H. 1971. U.S. Patent 3,610,731.

Shelton, J. C., F. K. Reinhart, and R. A. Logan. 1978. Appl. Opt. 17:2548–2555.

Stillman, G. E., L. W. Cook, N. Tabatabaie, G. E. Bulman, and V. M. Robbins. 1983. IEEE Trans. Electron. Devices ED-30:364.

Szoke, A., J. Goldhar, and N. A. Kurnit. 1969. Appl. Phys. Lett. 15:376.

Temkin, H., G. J. Dolan, R. A. Logan, R. F. Kazarinov, N. A. Olsson, and C. H. Henry. 1985. Appl. Phys. Lett. 46:105.

Tsang, W. T. 1981. Appl. Phys. Lett. 39:786.

Tsang, W. T., N. A. Olsson, and R. A. Logan. 1983. Appl. Phys. Lett. 42:650.

Tsang, W. T., N. A. Olsson, R. A. Logan, C. H. Henry, L. F. Johnson, J. E. Bowers, and J. Long. 1985. IEEE J. Quantum Electron. QE-21(6):519–526.

Wiener, J. S., D. A. B. Miller, D. S. Chemla, T. C. Damen, C. A. Burrus, T. H. Wood, A. C. Gossard, and W. Wiegmann. 1985. Appl. Phys. Lett. 47:1148.

Wood, T. H., C. A. Burrus, R. S. Tucker, J. S. Weiner, D. A. B. Miller, D. S. Chemla, T. C. Damen, A. C. Gossard, and W. Wiegmann. 1985. Electron. Lett. 21:693.

Woodall, J. M., H. Rupprecht, and G. D. Pettit. 1967. Solid-State Device Conf., June 19, 1967, Santa Barbara, Calif. (Abstracts reported in IEEE Trans. Electron. Devices ED-14:630.)

APPENDIX A:
CHARACTERISTICS
OF OPTICAL FIBERS

FIBER LOSS

Two parameters determine the usefulness of optical fibers in lightwave transmission. Both limit the maximum distance information can travel before it has to be regenerated using repeaters. The first is the propagation loss, which makes the signals weaker as they propagate down the fiber until they reach a point at which detection with a reasonable signal-to-noise ratio becomes a problem. The second is the dispersion of light in the fibers, which leads to a broadening of the lightwave pulses during propagation. This puts a combined limit on the data rate and distance of propagation. The linewidth of the laser source plays an important role in the dispersion-limited propagation, while the laser power launched in the fiber plays a crucial role in the absorption-limited regime. However, the input power to an optical fiber cannot be increased arbitrarily, even by staying below obvious limits of materials damage. In single-mode fibers especially, nonlinear interactions such as stimulated Brillouin and Raman scattering begin to become important at high laser intensities. These processes, which act to limit the maximum useful power injection into the fiber, can be used advantageously for in-line amplification of lightwave signals.

At present, the silica fiber losses have been reduced to minimum levels predicted by Rayleigh scattering, which, because of its λ^{-4} dependence, suggests that operation at longer wavelengths can yield even lower losses than the smallest loss seen in Figure 2. To exploit this possibility, a considerable amount of work is in progress to determine the best material systems that do not have intrinsic loss limits imposed by molecular vibrational frequencies of the constituents of the materials

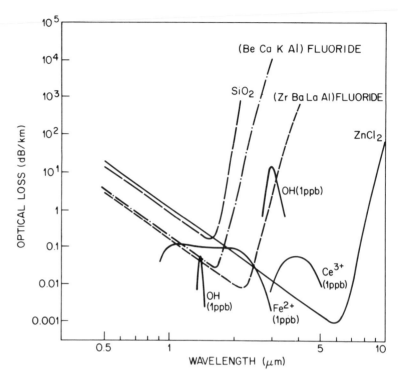

FIGURE A-1   Calculated spectral loss data for silica, sulfide, and fluoride fibers. Experimental data are also indicated.

or the impurities. Figure A-1 shows theoretical loss spectra for the silica, sulfide, and fluoride glasses (Lines, 1984). Silica fibers, as mentioned above, are already at or near their theoretical minimum loss limits of approximately 0.1–0.2 dB/km at 1.55 μm. Fluoride materials, for example, should show minimum loss approaching 10^{-2} dB/km at about 2.3 μm. The current losses (Tran et al., 1986; Yoshida, 1986), however, are approximately 0.7 dB/km at about 2.3 μm. The discrepancy of almost 2 orders of magnitude between the expected and the observed loss at 2.3 μm is probably the result of impurities, and can probably be reduced, much as the loss in silica fiber was reduced by more than 3 orders of magnitude between 1973 and 1983. Other materials, notably $ZnCl_2$, could have losses as small as 10^{-3} dB/km at 6.0 μm.

Although it is impossible to predict when the measured losses in practical fibers will come close to the expected values, it is interesting to speculate (Patel, 1981) about the impact of a 10^{-3}-dB/km loss for lightwave fibers. This could make possible a

transatlantic lightwave communication channel with no repeaters between the continental United States and Europe. If the
present division between the cost of the fiber cable and that of
the repeaters continues to hold for the longer wavelength fibers
and detectors and lasers, the cost of the transatlantic lightwave
system and all other long-distance systems can drop significantly. This reduction might further affect the balance between
satellite and lightwave communication for large bandwidth
information exchange across the Atlantic Ocean.

FIBER DISPERSION

Although loss characteristics of the current silica fibers are
relatively constant over a reasonably broad spectral range—for
example, covering a few hundred angstroms around 1.3 or 1.55
μm—the propagation group velocity changes significantly over
even such a narrow range of wavelengths. This dispersion in
group velocity has little or no effect on low-bit-rate transmission.
However, at high bit rates, the group velocity difference for
frequencies comprising the Fourier component of the light
pulse leads to a pulse broadening that limits the maximum fiber
span between repeaters. Chromatic dispersion, D, is a measure
of the pulse spreading and is defined as a differential of the
group delay t_g,

$$D = \frac{1}{L} \frac{dt_g}{d\lambda}$$

$$= \frac{1}{c} \frac{dn_g}{d\lambda}$$

$$= -\frac{\lambda}{c} \frac{d^2n}{d\lambda^2}, \tag{1}$$

where t_g is the propagation delay for a fiber of length L given by:

$$t_g = \frac{L}{v_g}, \tag{2}$$

where v_g is the group velocity and n_g is the group index given by:

$$n_g = \frac{c}{v_g}, \tag{3}$$

and n_g is a function of wavelength, in general, which leads to
nonzero chromatic dispersion, D. At approximately 1.3 μm in

silica fibers, $D = 0$ (see Figure 13), giving rise to a desirable situation of zero pulse broadening for a narrow linewidth laser input. In general, however, D is nonzero. By changing the dopants or the index profile of the fiber core and cladding, the zero dispersion point can be shifted to a limited extent (Gloge, 1971; Cohen et al., 1982) without significantly increasing the absorption losses.

The spectral width of the light pulse has two primary components. The first is the fundamental one that has its origin in the Fourier spectrum of the pulse, and this cannot be avoided. However, in practical situations, the lasers used for lightwave communication themselves possess spectral widths arising from multilongitudinal or other nonoptimal operation. For a typical multimode laser operating in the 1.3- or 1.55-μm region, linewidths as broad as 70–100 Å are not unusual, corresponding to laser oscillation on three longitudinal modes of the optical cavity of the semiconductor laser. For a single longitudinal-mode laser with a distributed feedback (DFB) grating integral to the laser, linewidths of the order of 1 Å are routine. Compared to these linewidths, the Fourier transform-limited spectral width for a 2-GHz/s bit rate is approximately 0.5 Å. Thus, the propagation of 2-GHz/s bit rate pulses from multimode and single-mode lasers will experience different dispersion-related limitations.

Figure 13 shows group velocity dispersion data for a single transverse-mode silica fiber plotted as a function of wavelength. The dispersion has been plotted in picoseconds of pulse broadening per kilometer of propagation and per nanometer of spectral width. The 1.3-μm low-loss window seen in Figure 13 for the silica fibers corresponds to a zero dispersion point of the fiber. Operating at the zero dispersion point avoids the problems of pulse broadening due to dispersion. The transatlantic lightwave system—TAT-8—due to be installed in the near future takes advantage of the zero dispersion point (Runge and Trischitta, 1984).

As seen from the spectral variation of the fiber loss, however, the lowest loss for the silica fiber occurs at a wavelength of 1.55 μm, where the dispersion is approximately 20 ps/km nm. At this wavelength, we would expect that at a 2-GHz/s bit rate, a practical single-mode distributed feedback laser pulse (linewidth ~1 Å) would broaden from an initial pulse width of 500 ps to about 750 ps when propagating through a 35-km fiber. The pulse from the multimode laser, on the other hand, would, for the same initial pulse width of 500 ps, broaden to about 7.5 ns going through the 35-km span, thus making communication impossible at this bit rate with a 35-km repeater span.

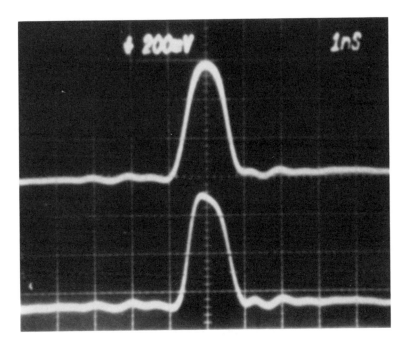

FIGURE A-2   Propagation of 1-ns laser pulses from a single-mode laser (linewidth, ~1 Å) at 1.55 μm through a single-mode fiber 35 km long. No detectable dispersion-induced broadening of the output pulse (top) is seen. (Bottom: input pulse.)

Figures A-2 and A-3 show (N. A. Olsson, personal communication) experimental demonstration of single-longitudinal versus multilongitudinal laser source injection into a fiber 35 km long. The pulse width is 1 ns at input, corresponding to a data rate of approximately 500 Mbit/s. Notice that the single-mode source pulse has no significant broadening at the output of the fiber. On the other hand, the multimode source pulse has broadened to about 10 ns, and the output pulse has three distinct peaks that correspond to each of the three longitudinal modes of the laser propagating at different velocities. In these cases, the loss-limited fiber span would have been $\gtrsim$ 200 km. Thus, in general, dispersion tends to limit the repeater spacing at high data rates.

The data representing records for longest path propagation as a function of the bit rate for a wavelength of 1.55 μm are shown (T. Li, personal communication) in Figure A-4. The loss-limited straight line corresponds to direct detection with a -45-dBm capability detector. The additional straight lines with larger negative slopes are drawn for 2-, 1-, and 0-Å laser

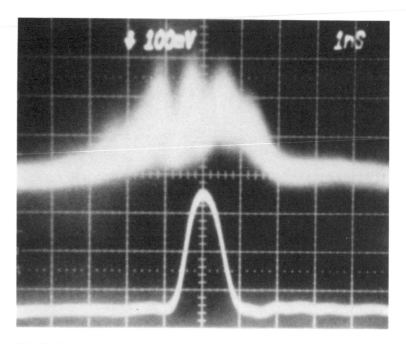

FIGURE A-3   Propagation of 1-ns pulses from a multilongitudinal mode laser at 1.55 μm through a single-mode fiber 35 km long (other experimental conditions are identical to those in Figure A-2). Laser line width is ~70 Å. Significant dispersion-induced broadening of the output pulse is seen. The breakup of the output pulse into three distinguishable components reflects the laser operation on three longitudinal modes, each one of which has a slightly different group velocity.

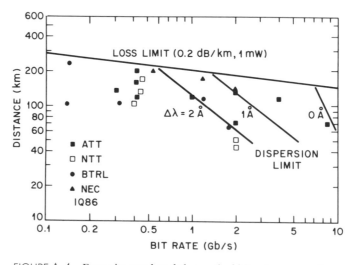

FIGURE A-4   Experimental and theoretical bit rate versus distance data.

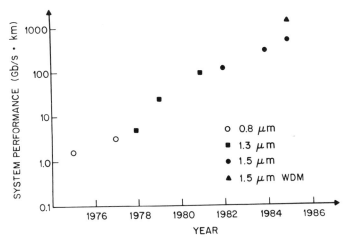

FIGURE A-5   Lightwave system performance (Gbit/s × km) as a function of time. (WDM corresponds to a 10-channel multiplex study.)

linewidths, which represent the dispersion-limited span maxima. Now we see that a loss of 10^{-3} dB/km in future fibers does not immediately portend 10,000-km repeater spacing if the fibers have finite dispersion. Nonlinear phenomena such as soliton propagation have to be invoked to compensate for the unacceptable pulse broadening that will accompany the longer repeater spans promised by ever-decreasing fiber losses. Finally, another way of measuring the figure of merit of a lightwave system is to calculate the product of the data rate (bits per second) and the maximum distance between repeaters (consistent with acceptable received bit error rate). Figure A-5 shows the performance (bit rate multiplied by the distance) of lightwave systems as a function of time, beginning in 1975. Rapid improvement has occurred since that time. (The WDM data point is for a 10-laser, 1.55-μm wavelength multiplex system described elsewhere in this paper.)

SOLITON PROPAGATION

Hasegawa and Tappert (1973) pointed out that intensity-dependent nonlinear effects in the index of refraction of an optical fiber, given by:

$$n = n_0 + \tfrac{1}{2}n_2 I, \qquad (4)$$

where n_0 is the refractive index of the fiber at low intensities, I is the optical field intensity, and n_2 is the nonlinear index, can be used for compensating the effect of chromatic dispersion, D.

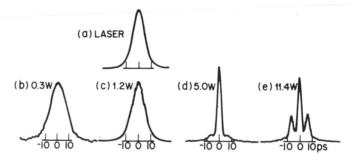

FIGURE A-6   Soliton propagation in a single-mode fiber of length equal to a half-soliton period. (a) This shows the laser pulse as it is launched into the fiber. (b) $P = 0.3$ W. Negligible nonlinear effects seen; only dispersive broadening takes place. (c) $P = 1.2$ W. Output pulse width narrows to the same as that for input pulse corresponding to the fundamental soliton propagation. (d) $P = 5.0$ W. Output pulse narrowed to minimum width corresponding to half period behavior of $n = 2$ solitons. (e) $P = 11.4$ W. First well-resolved splitting of the output pulse corresponding to $n = 3$ solitons. (Note that the threefold splitting in the these autocorrelation traces correspond to a twofold splitting of the pulse itself.)

Even though n_2 has a very small numeric value, given by $n_2 \approx 3.2 \times 10^{-16}$ cm^2 W^{-1}, the long propagation lengths possible in low-loss fibers and the small core diameter of the single-mode fibers that yield high optical field intensities make it possible to see the effect of the nonlinear index. For example, a laser pulse with a power of 1 mW in a typical single-mode fiber produces an intensity $I. \geq 10^3$ Wcm^{-2}. Hasegawa and Tappert's studies showed that under suitable conditions, stable pulses that maintain their shape and width can be propagated in low-loss, single-mode fibers. These shape-maintaining pulses, called envelope solitons, result from an interplay between the normal dispersion of the fiber, which would tend to broaden the pulses, and the nonlinear index, which tends to sharpen them. A stable soliton pulse in a fiber has a hyperbolic secant shape.

In several elegant experiments, Mollenauer and his colleagues have shown the existence of such soliton propagation at modest values of injected laser power (Mollenauer et al., 1980). Figure A-6 shows the results of one of the early experiments to demonstrate the propagation of solitons in approximately 700-m-long single-mode fibers. The lowest input power autocorrelation trace of the output is for $P_{in} \sim 0.3$ W, for which a pulse broadening occurs because of the chromatic dispersion of approximately 16 ps/km nm. For input power above this value, a monotonic narrowing of the output pulse was observed; at $P_{in} \sim$ 1.2 W the output pulse width mirrored the input pulse width and reached a minimum of 2 ps at $P_{in} \sim$ 5.0 W. At higher powers, the output pulse shows splitting caused by higher order solitons. For this experiment, the length of the fiber was half a soliton characteristic period, z_0, defined by:

$$z_0 = 0.322 \pi^2 \frac{c}{\lambda^2} \frac{\tau^2}{D}, \qquad (5)$$

where τ is the full width at the half-intensity maxima of the pulse. For longer fiber lengths, soliton shape is no longer preserved at all points along the fiber but is recovered at the end of each soliton period. This assumes that the characteristic absorption length, $1/\alpha$, of the fiber is much larger than the soliton period.

In a practical system for optical fiber lengths (i.e., repeater spacings) much greater than the absorption length, the soliton can no longer be preserved without periodic "in-line" amplification of the soliton intensity (Hasegawa and Kodama, 1982; Hasegawa, 1984). Such amplification can take advantage of Raman gain in silica fibers when laser radiation at high frequency and relatively high power is injected (see Figure A-7). The Raman gain overcomes the distributed loss of the fiber, as well as local loss due to insertion of the directional coupler into the fiber path. Such in-line amplification may have advantages even when soliton propagation is not used (Hegarty et al., 1985). Further, the use of semiconductor lasers as amplifiers has also been explored as a way to compensate for the fiber loss in a coherent lightwave communication system. Olsson has shown that in such a configuration, there is essentially no penalty incurred in the bit error rate (Hegarty et al., 1985).

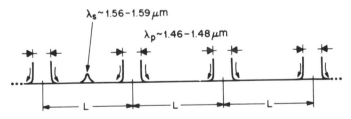

$\lambda_s \sim 1.56 - 1.59 \, \mu m$

$\lambda_p \sim 1.46 - 1.48 \, \mu m$

FIGURE A-7 In-line Raman amplification for an all-optical lightwave system. At "repeaters" spaced by L, continuous wave laser diodes inject power (at λ_p) into the optical fiber in both directions (through wavelength-dependent directional couplers) for the Raman gain to compensate for the loss experienced by data pulses (λ_s).

TABLE A-1   Design Parameters for a Single-Channel Soliton-Based Lightwave System

Parameter	Value
Input power	3.0 mW
In-line amplifier separation	50 km
Pulse width	22.6 ps
Data rate	4.4 Gbit/s
Total distance	6,600 km

The in-line optical amplification avoids the multitude of complexities associated with the conventional repeaters that rely on optical-to-electronic-to-optical signal conversions. These various conversions and the electronic paths themselves can limit the bit rate. Further, for the wavelength division multiplexing scheme (Olsson et al., 1985), the conventional repeaters become unduly complex when we try to take advantage of the enormous bandwidth of lightwave communications by multiplexing tens of individual wavelengths on a single fiber. For example, each of the repeaters would need the optical demultiplexer and the optical multiplexer together with one electronic channel for each of the wavelength division multiplexed lightwave channels.

A parametric investigation of the usefulness of soliton propagation systems in conjunction with in-line Raman amplification in the fiber itself yields (Mollenauer et al., 1986) products of bit rate and distance approximating 30,000 GHz-km for a single-fiber system and 300,000 GHz-km for a 24-channel WDM system, as shown in Table A-1. Signal laser powers of the order of ≤ 10 mW are sufficient with pump powers of the order of a few hundred milliwatts at in-line amplifier "repeater" lengths of approximately 50 km. Although these numbers represent extrapolations from observed soliton propagation, they could nonetheless be possible options for future ultrahigh-performance lightwave systems.

REFERENCES

Cohen, L. G., W. L. Mammel, and S. J. Jamg. 1982. Electron. Lett. 18:1023–1024.

Gloge, D. 1971. Appl. Opt. 10:2252 and 2442.

Hasegawa, A. 1984. Appl. Opt. 23:3302–3309.

Hasegawa, A., and Y. Kodama. 1982. Opt. Lett. 7:287.

Hasegawa, A., and F. Tappert. 1973. Appl. Phys. Lett. 23:142.

Hegarty, J., N. A. Olsson, and L. Goldner. 1985. Electron. Lett. 21:290–292.

Lines, M. E. 1984. J. Appl. Phys. 55:4058.

Mollenauer, L. F., R. H. Stolen, and J. P. Gordon. 1980. Phys. Rev. Lett. 45:1095.

Mollenauer, L. F., J. P. Gordon, and M. N. Islam. 1986. IEEE J. Quantum Electron. QE-22:157–173.

Olsson, N. A., J. Hegarty, R. A. Logan, L. F. Johnson, K. L. Walker, L. G. Cohen, B. L. Kasper, and J. C. Campbell. 1985. Electron. Lett. 31:105.

Patel, C. K. N. 1981. Soc. Photo-Opt. Inst. Eng. 266:22.

Runge, P. K., and P. R. Trischitta. 1984. IEEE Selected Areas Commun. SAC-2:784–793.

Tran, D. C., K. Levin, M. Burk, C. Fister, and W. Broer. 1986. Proc. SPIE Symp. Infrared Optical Material and Fiber 618:48.

Yoshida, S. 1986. Paper presented at the North Atlantic Treaty Organization Advanced Research Workshop on Halide Glasses for Infrared Fibers, March.

APPENDIX B:
DETECTORS IN OPTICAL
COMMUNICATIONS

PIN PHOTODETECTORS AND PIN-FET RECEIVERS

State-of-the-art PIN photodiodes in the $\lambda = 1.3–1.6$-μm range consist of mesa or planar $In_{0.53}Ga_{0.47}As$ pn junctions, grown lattice matched to InP substrates, with very low doped n layers ($<5 \times 10^{15}$ cm^{-3}) to achieve the required low capacitance ($\lesssim 0.5$ pF) (Pearsall and Pollack, 1985). These devices are typically operated at low reverse bias voltage (<10 V) with dark currents of a few nanoamperes and external quantum efficiencies of 60–70 percent at $\lambda = 1.55$ and 1.3 μm. These detectors, in combination with a GaAs field-effect transistor (FET) front-end amplifier, have found wide use in fiber-optic receivers at data rates up to 400 Mbit/s. Experimental tests and theoretical evaluations have indeed shown that in this bit rate range, the use of state-of-the-art InP/GaInAs avalanche photodiodes (APDs) in place of the PIN photodiode in receivers yields a typical improvement in sensitivity of 1 or 2 dB. On the other hand, the APD technology is much more demanding and costly than the PIN technology, and high-reliability planar 1.3- to 1.6-μm APDs have not yet been demonstrated. These considerations explain why the PIN-FET combination has been the most widely used in receivers at data rates of less than about 400 Mbit/s (Forrest, 1985).

The minimum noise that an FET front-end amplifier can achieve in a photoreceiver is proportional to C_T/g_m. C_T is the total capacitance, which contains contributions from the detector, the FET, and parasitics (interconnects); and g_m is the FET transconductance. C_T should be minimized to maximize the receiver sensitivity. The latter quantity is defined as the optical power required to achieve a bit error rate of 10^{-9}. The best PIN-receiver sensitivities have been achieved using a hybrid combination of a mesa GaInAs PIN and a GaAs semiconductor field-effect transistor with $C_T = 0.5$ pF. This sensitivity is -42 dB/m at $\lambda = 1.3$ μm for a bit rate of 500 Mbit/s (Forrest, 1985).

HETEROJUNCTION AVALANCHE PHOTODIODES

Simple homojunction $Ga_{0.47}In_{0.53}As$ photodiodes cannot be operated as low-noise avalanche detectors because the dark current becomes prohibitively large because of Zener tunneling across the band gap at voltages at which impact ionization sets in (Pearsall and Pollack, 1985). This important fact, completely overlooked by proponents of the homojunction approach, is a consequence of the small gap (0.73 eV) and small electron effective mass in this alloy. This finding, first reported in 1980, clearly demonstrated the need for suitable heterojunction APDs (Pearsall and Pollack, 1985).

An important step in this direction was the proposal and 1979 demonstration of an APD that consisted of an InP *pn* junction grown next to a GaInAs(P) layer. To minimize the Zener tunneling in this device, the maximum electric field of the *pn* junction is located in the InP wide gap layers where the avalanche takes place, and the GaInAs(P) layer absorbs the infrared photons (Figure B-1). Hence, the name SAM (separate

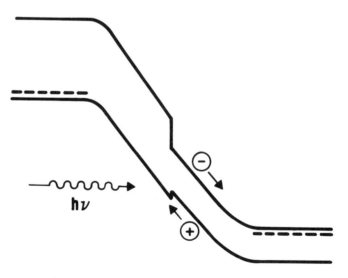

FIGURE B-1   Band diagram of an SAM (separate absorption and multiplication) avalanche photodiode

absorption and multiplication) APD is given to this structure (Pearsall and Pollack, 1985). This device achieves good gains (10–20) and low dark currents (nearly 50 nA), provided the doping and thickness of the avalanche region are carefully tailored and controlled.

However, a serious problem of this structure was discovered shortly after the device was demonstrated. When a $Ga_{0.47}In_{0.53}As$ absorbing layer is used, photogenerated holes, in the process of drifting into the InP layer, tend to pile up at the heterojunction interface. This effect produces a long tail (tens of microseconds in the worst cases) in the pulse response, making it impossible to use these devices at high bit rates. Researchers at the AT&T Bell Laboratories recently solved this problem when they introduced an intermediate quaternary GaInAsP grading layer between the absorbing GaInAs layer and the InP avalanche region (Pearsall and Pollack, 1985) and, alternatively, introduced a chirped $InP/Ga_{0.47}In_{0.53}As$ superlattice that simulates a graded gap GaInAsP layer (Figure B-2) (Capasso, 1985). Such pseudoquaternary alloys represent a good example of band-gap engineering and should find applications in other optoelectronic devices as well, such as graded-index separate confinement heterostructure (GRINSCH) InP/GaInAs lasers.

High-performance InP/GaInAs SAM APDs with one or two intermediate grading layers have recently been developed by Holden and others (Holden et al., 1985). These devices have dark current gains of 60 and gain-bandwidth products of 60 GHz and have captured all of the world records in receiver sensitivity experiments at bit rates exceeding 400 Mbit/s (Kasper, 1986). For example, recent tests at 4 and 8 Gbit/s at $\lambda = 1.5$ μm with a GaAs FET front-end have yielded receiver sensitivities of -31.2 and -26 dBm, respectively. The best values obtained at 420 and 2 Gbit/s are instead -44 and -36.6 dBm. These sensitivities are 5–10 dB better than those achieved with PIN photodiodes. To obtain an even higher sensitivity, the dark current should be further reduced, and the electron/hole ionization rate ratio should be increased (in InP SAM APDs, $\beta/\alpha = 3$).

The reduction of the dark current should produce a large sensitivity increase compared to PIN-FET receivers at low bit rates (<400 Mbits) as well. Such a reduction can be achieved by means of the recently demonstrated Hi-Lo SAM APD (Capasso et al., 1984a). In this device, a thin, heavily doped region is introduced in the lightly doped InP avalanche layer so that the electric field drops to a low value in the InP and GaInAs regions immediately adjacent to the heterointerface. In this structure,

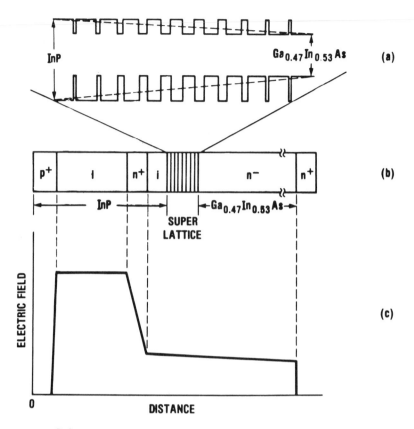

FIGURE B-2   Band diagram (a), device structure (b), and electric-field profile (c) of an SAM avalanche photodiode with chirped superlattice to eliminate carrier pileup at the InP/GaInAs interface.

the electric field at the heterointerface is significantly smaller than in a conventional SAM APD, thus reducing the dark current to lower values. This effect was demonstrated in AlIn-As/GaInAs Hi-Lo SAM APDs grown by molecular beam epitaxy (MBE) and in InP/GaInAs Hi-Lo SAM APDs grown by liquid-phase epitaxy.

SAM APDs have also been studied extensively in AlInAs/GaInAs alloys. A potential advantage of this combination is that the band discontinuities are more favorably aligned for high-speed operation. In fact, AlInAs/GaInAs SAM APDs without intermediate grading layers have demonstrated a speed of response comparable to that of InP/GaInAs SAM APDs with grading layers (Capasso et al., 1984b). The quality of the AlInAs must be improved, however, before these detectors can become a real challenge for InP-based APDs.

ADVANCED AVALANCHE PHOTODIODES AND
SOLID-STATE PHOTOMULTIPLIERS

The multiplication noise of an avalanche photodiode is known to increase strongly, at a given value of the gain M, as the ratio of the electron/hole ionization coefficients $\kappa = \alpha/\beta$ approaches unity. In fact, it can be shown that in this limit, the APD noise is proportional to M^3, whereas in the opposite ideal limit, in which only one carrier can ionize, the noise increases as a function of M^2 (McIntyre, 1966). Most III-V alloys, including InP used in SAM APDs, have an ionization rate ratio (α/β or β/α) in the range from 1 to 3, and as such are unsuitable to achieve the low noise performance of Si APDs at shorter wavelengths (in Si, $\alpha/\beta \gtrsim 20$).

Research has concentrated on multilayer structures capable of artificially enhancing α/β using material systems with α approximately equal to β. These efforts have led Capasso (1985) to the concept of a solid-state photomultiplier. In 1981 a group at Bell Laboratories showed that in an MBE-grown AlGaAs/GaAs quantum well APD the α/β ratio is enhanced by a factor of 4 over the bulk value for α/β GaAs (Capasso, 1985). This effect is partially due to the difference between the conduction and valence band discontinuities. At the University of Michigan, more recent extensive work on such structures has shown the above effect for a greater range of layer thicknesses (Juang et al., 1985). A potential problem in this structure is that the pileup of carriers in the quantum wells may deteriorate the pulse response. Recently, however, Mohammed and colleagues showed this is not a problem and demonstrated response times of less than 200 ps in AlInAs/GaInAs quantum well APDs (Mohammed et al., 1986). This is due to hot electron effects and tunneling through the barriers.

Another structure designed to enhance the α/β ratio is a PIN APD with a graded gap in the i region. Electrons, which move toward lower gap regions than holes, "see" a lower ionization energy, and this effect enhances the α/β ratio (Figure B-3). Ionization ratios of 5 to 7 have been demonstrated in an AlGaAs prototype structure (Capasso, 1985).

Yet another approach is the channeling APD in which the α/β ratio is enhanced by spatially separating electrons and holes in materials of different band gaps (Capasso, 1985). This is done using an interdigitated npnp lateral structure (Figure B-4). This new depletion and detection scheme has several other advantages (experimentally demonstrated), such as the extremely low capacitance that is independent of the sensitive area of the detector and the large volume of depleted material. Interest-

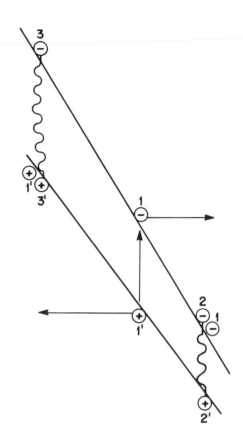

FIGURE B-3 Band diagram of high-field region of a graded gap avalanche photodiode. The 1-1' electron-hole pair initiates avalanche multiplication as follows: Electron 1 creates by impact ionization the electron-hole pair 2-2' in the lower gap region. Hole 1' creates the electron-hole pair 3-3' in the higher gap region. Thus, the electron has a lower ionization energy than the hole.

ingly, the channeling detector concept has found important applications in nuclear physics as a position-sensitive drift chamber to detect high-energy particles (Gatti and Rehak, 1984).

Probably the most promising of these structures for optical communications is the staircase avalanche photodiode, which is the solid-state analog of a photomultiplier (Capasso, 1985). The structure consists of a graded gap superlattice low-doped layer sandwiched between a p^+ and n^+ layer. When a reverse bias is applied, the sawtooth potential profile is converted in a potential staircase. The materials are chosen in such a way that the magnitude of the step (conduction band discontinuity) is greater than the gap after the step, and the valence band step is negligible (Figure B-5). Electrons impact-ionize only at the steps because only there does their kinetic energy exceed the band gap, whereas holes do not ionize. Capasso has shown theoretically that the excess noise factor F for such a structure is practically unity, similar to a phototube (Capasso, 1985). No other type of APD, including an ideal conventional one in which only one type of carrier can ionize, has this unique property. In fact, until recently, the lower theoretical limit for F at high gains was thought to be 2. One additional advantage of the staircase APD is the low-voltage operation (≈ 5 V for a gain of ≈ 30). The materials that are investigated for this application are HgCdTe and AlGaAs/GaSb grown by MBE. Experimental demonstrations have not yet been reported. Clearly, the staircase detector has the potential for achieving unprecedented receiver sensitivities at both high and low bit rates, provided one can minimize the dark current of the device.

Another approach to the solid-state photomultiplier is based on a recently discovered avalanche multiplication mechanism (impact ionization across the band-edge discontinuity (Capasso et al., 1986). In suitably designed superlattice structures, hot carriers in the barrier layers can collide with carriers confined or dynamically stored in the wells and impact-ionize them out across the band-edge discontinuity (Figure B-6). In this ionization effect, only one type of carrier is created, so that the positive feedback is eliminated, leading to the possibility of a quiet avalanche with small excess noise. A multistage graded gap avalanche photodiode based on this concept has been demonstrated, and it exhibits a near single-carrier-type multiplication, similar to a photomultiplier (Allam et al., 1987).

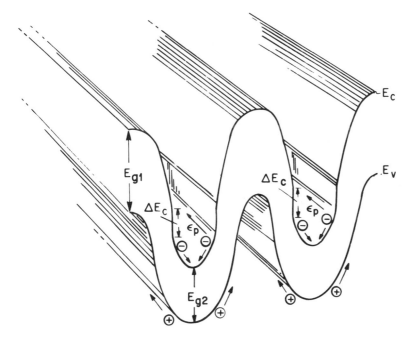

FIGURE B-4   Band diagram of the channeling avalanche photodiode.

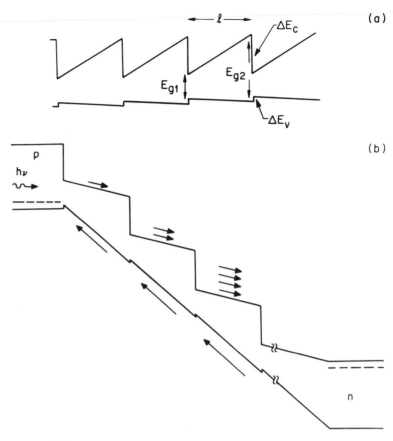

FIGURE B-5   Band diagram of the staircase solid-state photomultiplier. (a) shows the unbiased graded multilayer region, and (b) shows the complete staircase detector under bias. The arrows in the valence band indicate that the holes do not impact-ionize; hole multiplication due to electron-initiated impact ionization is not shown for simplicity.

Recently, an SAM APD with an Si-Ge superlattice absorbing layer and a Si multiplication region has been demonstrated (Temkin et al., 1986). To maximize absorption without degrading high-speed operation, the device has a waveguide geometry (lateral illumination) (Figure B-7). The device has potential for achieving the low multiplication noise of silicon at long wavelengths, but part of this advantage is offset by the relatively large coupling losses and other technological difficulties associated with the lateral illumination. One of the most interesting applications of this device is for integrated optics.

At compositions such that the spin-orbit splitting approximately equals the band-gap in certain alloys ($Al_xGa_{1-x}Sb$,

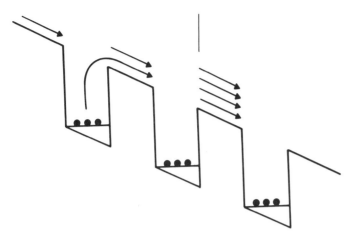

FIGURE B-6   Band diagram of solid-state photomultiplier based on impact ionization across the band-edge discontinuity of carriers stored in the wells.

$Hg_{1-x}Cd_xTe$), the ionization rates β/α ratio attains a large value (10–20) because of the near-zero momentum transfer in the ionizing collisions of holes (resonance impact-ionization) (Capasso, 1985). These compositions correspond to band gaps $\lambda_g \approx$ 1.3–1.5 μm and thus may be suitable for avalanche detectors for communication systems. HgCdTe appears particularly promising from this point of view because the dark currents are much

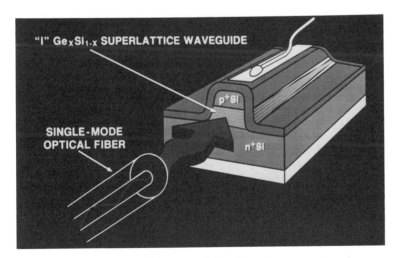

FIGURE B-7   Schematic diagram of Ge_x-Si_{1-x} long-wavelength waveguide superlattice avalanche PIN photodiode.

lower than the corresponding AlGaSb alloy of the same gap. Société Anonyme de Télécommunications in France has already developed HgCdTe PIN detectors at $\lambda = 1.3$ μm with dark currents of approximately 1 nA and plans to have a working low-noise 1.3-μm APD using the above resonance effect in the near future.

PHOTOCONDUCTORS

In recent years, $Ga_{0.47}In_{0.53}As$ photoconductors have attracted considerable attention as possible alternatives to PIN and avalanche detectors in the 1.3–1.6-μm wavelength regions. The best results so far obtained at bit rates of 1 Gbit/s are 1 or 2 dB lower in sensitivity than the best PIN-FET receivers (Chen et al., 1984). Extensive theoretical analyses at the AT&T Bell Laboratories have shown that in the above wavelength range and at bit rates ranging from 500 Mbit/s to 2 Gbit/s, the photoconductor can, at best, match the performance of a PIN in a receiver but never do better than an APD (Forrest, 1985). On the other hand, the photoconductor has advantages of very low voltage operation and easy fabrication technology. These features may

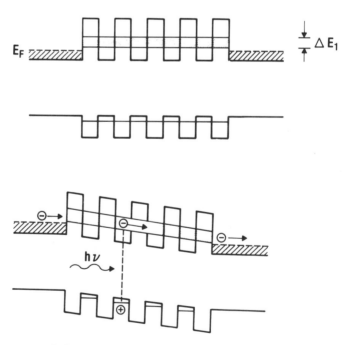

FIGURE B-8   Band diagram of superlattice photoconductor; shown is the effective mass filtering mechanism.

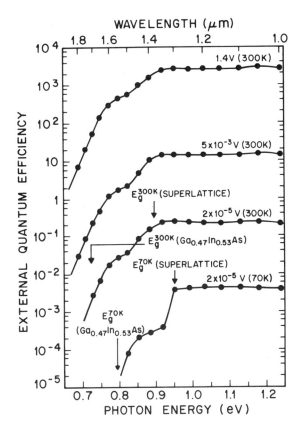

FIGURE B-9   Current gain in an effective mass filter detector.

be attractive for applications in which one is willing to trade performance against cost, such as local area networks. In addition, the lateral geometry makes the photoconductor particularly attractive for monolithic integration with an FET.

Recently, Capasso and coworkers (1985) have demonstrated a new type of photoconductor called an effective mass filter. This structure consists of a superlattice with thin layers (30-Å barrier and 30-Å wells) and achieves high gain and low noise at very low voltages (<0.2 V) using the large difference between the tunneling rates of electrons and holes through the superlattice barriers (Figures B-8 and B-9). Although the most recently demonstrated device is slow, another variety of effective mass filter that uses miniband conduction of electrons rather than phonon-assisted tunneling has potential for high-speed, low-noise, and low-voltage operation. These features may make such detectors attractive for optical communication systems, particularly at wavelengths beyond 1.5 μm.

REFERENCES

Allam, J., F. Capasso, K. Alavi, and A. Y. Cho. In press. Proceedings of the GaAs Symposium. Las Vegas, Nev.

Capasso, F. 1985. The physics of avalanche photodiodes. P. 1 in Semiconductors and Semimetals, Vol. 22, Lightwave Communications Technology: Part A, Material Growth Technologies, W. T. Tsang, ed. New York: Academic Press.

Capasso, F., A. Y. Cho, and P. W. Foy. 1984a. Electron. Lett. 20:635.

Capasso, F., B. Kasper, K. Alavi, A. Y. Cho, and J. M. Parsey. 1984b. Appl. Phys. Lett. 44:1027.

Capasso, F., J. Allam, A. Y. Cho, K. Mohammed, R. J. Malik, A. L. Hutchinson, and D. Sivco. 1986. Appl. Phys. Lett. 48:1294.

Chen, C. Y., B. L. Kasper, and H. M. Cox. 1984. Appl. Phys. Lett. 44:1142.

Forrest, S. R. 1985. P. 329 in Semiconductors and Semimetals, Vol. 22, Lightwave Communications Technology: Part A, Material Growth Technologies, W. T. Tsang, ed. New York: Academic Press.

Gatti, E., and P. Rehak. 1984. Nuclear Instr. Methods 225:608.

Holden, W. S., J. C. Campbell, J. F. Ferguson, A. G. Dentai, and Y. K. Jhee. 1985. Electron. Lett. 22:886.

Juang, F. Y., U. Das, Y. Nashimoto, and P. K. Bhattacharya. 1985. Appl. Phys. Lett. 47:972.

Kasper, B. L. 1986. P. 119 in Technical Digest of the Optical Fiber Communications Conference. Atlanta, Ga.

McIntyre, R. J. 1966. IEEE Trans. Electron. Devices ED-13:164.

Mohammed, K., F. Capasso, J. Allam, A. Y. Cho, and A. L. Hutchinson. 1986. Appl. Phys. Lett. 47:597.

Pearsall, T. P., and M. A. Pollack. 1985. P. 174 in Semiconductors and Semimetals, Vol. 22, Lightwave Communications Technology: Part A, Material Growth Technologies, W. T. Tsang, ed. New York: Academic Press.

Temkin, H., T. P. Pearsall, J. C. Bean, R. A. Logan, and S. Luryi. 1986. Appl. Phys. Lett. 48:963.

APPENDIX C:
COHERENT SYSTEM
EXPERIMENT

Conventional direct-detection lightwave receivers are limited in their performance by thermal noise. The only way to circumvent this problem is to amplify the signal without adding excess noise. One way to achieve this amplification is by heterodyne gain: The incoming optical signal is mixed with a local oscillator, and the beat signal, which contains the information, is multiplied by the local oscillator. Such systems, using a local oscillator, are called coherent systems. The principle is illustrated in Figure C-1, which shows the improvement in receiver sensitivity for a 150-Mbit/s coherent system by increasing the local oscillator power (N. A. Olsson, personal communication). As the local oscillator power is increased, the receiver sensitivity approaches the fundamental shot noise limit. However, because of nonideal components, such as the quantum efficiency of the detectors, the ultimate shot noise limit is hard to reach.

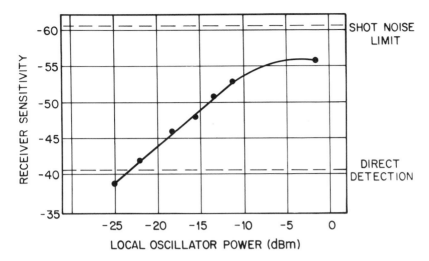

FIGURE C-1   Sensitivity improvement with coherent detection at a bit rate of 150 Mbit/s.

The coherent lightwave system experiment described here used differential phase shift keying (DPSK) at data rates of 400 Mbit/s and 1 Gbit/s and a transmission distance of 150 km. The system is depicted in Figure C-2 (Linke et al., 1986). The transmitter and local oscillator lasers are external cavity lasers. Phase modulation of the optical carrier was achieved with a titanium-diffused $LiNbO_3$ waveguide phase modulator (Schmidt and Cross, 1978). The modulator had an insertion loss of 1.8 dB and required a modulation voltage of 8.5 V peak to peak for a 180-degree phase shift. After transmission through 150 km of fiber with a transmission loss of 39.6 dB, the transmitted signal is mixed with the local oscillator in a 3-dB fiber coupler. The balanced-mixer dual-detector receiver efficiently uses the available local oscillator and signal power and suppresses any excess amplitude noise in the local oscillator. The equalized bandwidth of the high-impedance front end was more than 3.5 GHz. The intermediate-frequency (IF) signal was processed in a delay line discriminator, and part of the IF signal was used in a feedback circuit that frequency-locked the local oscillator laser to the incoming data signal. The system was evaluated by measuring the bit-error rate as a function of the received power. In both cases the error rate could be decreased to arbitrarily low levels (measured down to 1×10^{-10}) by increasing the received power. The absence of an error floor is the absolute proof of the spectral purity and low phase noise of the external cavity lasers

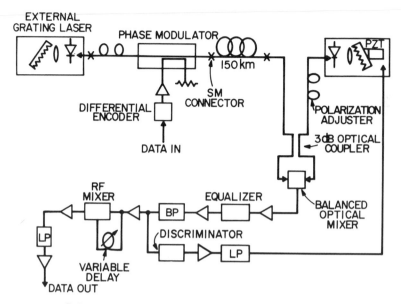

FIGURE C-2 Experimental setup for coherent detection lightwave demonstration.

used. The measured receiver sensitivity at 400 Mbit/s and 1 Gbit/s was −55.3 and −44 dBm, respectively. In the ideal shot noise limited case, DPSK modulation requires 21 photons per bit for a 1×10^{-9} error rate. The measured system performance was 6.4 and 11 dB from this theoretical limit at 400 Mbit/s and 1 Gbit/s, respectively. Part of the discrepancy is accounted for by the thermal noise of the receiver, and by the less-than-unity quantum efficiency of the photodetectors. In spite of the deviation from the ideal shot noise limit, the measured receiver sensitivities are the best reported for the respective data rate and are about six times better than the best reported direct detection sensitivities. This coherent system experiment is the first gigabit-per-second system and the first time a coherent system has outperformed the direct detection counterpart in transmission distance.

REFERENCES

Linke, R. A., B. L. Kasper, N. A. Olsson, and R. C. Alferness. 1986. Electron. Lett. 22:30–31.
Schmidt, R. V., and P. C. Cross. 1978. Opt. Lett. 2:45–47.

Lasers in Medicine

Rodney Perkins, M.D.

In nature, periodic mutation creates new life-forms and moves the species to new levels of performance and being. Similarly, from time to time in human endeavors, mutative cerebration provides important new concepts that we can then refine and develop into processes that we hope will enrich the human condition.

The laser is such a type of contribution. Its impact is already widespread in science, communication, industry, and medicine. This impact will grow rapidly as we better understand its nature, develop permutations, and integrate both basic and advanced forms closely with other core technologies to produce hybrids that can satisfy as yet unknown needs.

LIGHT IN MEDICINE

The use of the laser in medicine and surgery has a relatively short pedigree of less than two decades. Although the range of laser radiation extends both below and above the visible portion of the electromagnetic spectrum, that radiation is, in a sense, only a special form of light. The use of other forms of light in medicine has a longer history. There is documentation that the ancient Egyptians recognized and used the therapeutic power of light as long as 6,000 years ago (Figure 1). Patches of depigmented skin, now referred to as vitiligo, were cosmetically undesirable. Egyptian healers reportedly crushed a plant similar to presentday parsley and rubbed the affected areas with the crushed leaves. Exposure to the sun's radiation produced a severe form of sunburn only in the treated areas. The erythema

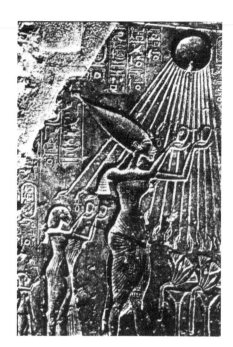

FIGURE 1   The ancient
Egyptians recognized many
beneficial qualities of solar
radiation. Photograph by
Glenn Calderhead.

subsided, leaving hyperpigmentation in the previously depigmented areas.

In Europe in the late eighteenth and early nineteenth centuries, at the height of the Industrial Revolution, a myriad of factories and industrial plants spewed smoke into the atmosphere, filtering out many of the beneficial components of the sun's rays. Deprivation of ultraviolet radiation contributed to calcium deficiency in the main skeletal bones, leading to the characteristic deformity known as rickets. The much more insidious and fatal pulmonary tuberculosis was also prevalent. It was found that sunlight helped alleviate the symptoms of these diseases, and so sanitariums sprang up all over Europe, especially in Great Britain and Switzerland. They were usually located on higher ground or by the sea, because this seemed to increase the efficacy of the therapy. We now know that pure air filters out fewer of the beneficial components of solar radiation.

In the late nineteenth century, the Danish scientist Nils Finsen used a quartz-and-water cooling system to extract the ultraviolet from both solar and man-made arc-lamp radiation to treat various skin conditions, such as vitiligo and psoriasis, a scaly overproduction in areas of skin. The significance of Finsen's work was that, for the first time, an artificial light source was being used therapeutically.

Sixty years later, only a quarter of a century ago, a light source more powerful than the sun was developed by Theodore H. Maiman at the Hughes Research Laboratories in Malibu, California, heralding a new era in phototherapy. Maiman's laser used a ruby crystal to produce its intense deep red beam. Other lasers using different media soon emerged. In 1960, Ali Javan created the helium-neon gas laser, first emitting in the infrared part of the spectrum and a year later in the important red line. A year later Peter A. Franken demonstrated that certain crystalline materials could effectively double the frequency of an incident beam. The year 1964 was a prolific year for laser development and yielded an outstanding harvest of lasers used in clinical medicine. C. Kumar N. Patel introduced the carbon dioxide (CO_2) gas laser, which produced an invisible beam in the far infrared. Another invisible laser in the near infrared, the neodymium yttrium-aluminum garnet (Nd:YAG) was contributed by Guesic, Marcos, and Van Uitert. The argon gas laser emitting in the visible blue-green spectrum was demonstrated by William Bridges. Since then, literally thousands of substances have been used to produce laser energy.

However, those first few that appeared so close together, in general, have remained until today the most popularly used lasers in clinical medicine and surgery (Plate 4). Maiman's ruby laser, although still occasionally used in some dermatological applications, is no longer in common medical use. The helium-neon laser is mainly used as an aiming beam for the invisible infrared CO_2 and Nd:YAG lasers. The argon laser is used extensively in ophthalmology and dermatology and less so in otology, neurosurgery, urology, and gynecology. Both infrared lasers, the Nd:YAG and particularly the CO_2, have found a variety of clinical applications. The CO_2 laser has been used to vaporize tissue in almost every specialty, whereas the Nd:YAG laser has been used primarily for tissue coagulation in gastroenterology and urology. A specialized short-pulse, high peak power Nd:YAG laser has been used effectively in ophthalmology after cataract surgery.

Frequency-doubled lasers were used only experimentally until a higher power laser was made possible by using doubling crystals of potassium titanyl phosphate (KTP) developed by J. Bierlein at Du Pont. The laser that resulted from doubling the Nd:YAG with KTP—called the KTP/532 laser—began clinical use in 1983 and is now being applied in a wide variety of surgical specialties.

MINIMALLY INVASIVE SURGERY

Why is the laser used in medicine, and why is its use increasing? Some answers can be found by looking at a few of the universal changes occurring in medicine. Economic, political, and sociological factors in our society frequently affect the disposition of scientific discovery, just as scientific and technological progress influences broad changes in the nontechnical spheres of human activity. These factors are Newtonian in the sense that actions in one sphere of activity have a direct influence on actions in other spheres.

In the past decade, there has been a growing trend toward a less invasive style of surgical intervention. This style is characterized by achieving a maximal treatment effect with minimal damage to surrounding and overlying normal structures and is termed minimally invasive surgery, or MIS.

The trend toward MIS is being driven by a multiplicity of factors. High-technology diagnostic devices, such as computerized axial tomography, magnetic resonance imaging, as well as sophisticated optical devices in the form of flexible fiber-optic endoscopes and intravascular catheters, have enhanced our ability to identify disease processes early and locate them accurately. Generally, the earlier a tumor or growth can be identified, the more responsive it is to therapy by a minimally invasive technique.

Human psychology is also part of this changing equation. Everyone has an inborn fear of standard invasive surgical procedures. Given an equivalent surgical outcome, we will almost always choose a less invasive procedure. The increase in patient consumerism, coupled with rapid and widespread transmission of information on new MIS procedures through video and popular print media, also fuels this trend.

Economics exerts a strong influence on the trend toward MIS. These procedures are cost-effective to insurers, corporations, and the government, since most are done on an outpatient basis. This results in reduced cost, lower morbidity, and less time away from work. Even when MIS techniques are used as an adjunct to more invasive surgical approaches, reduced destruction of tissue frequently leads to quicker recovery with a shortened, lower cost hospitalization.

The laser is an integral part of this trend toward MIS. It is well suited to MIS because it can create precision surgical effects at a distance. Laser energy can be transmitted through endoscopic devices passed through the body's natural orifices, or it can be

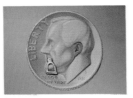

PLATE 5 (Above) The stapes bone is approximately the same length as the word *God* on a dime.

PLATE 6 (Right) The stapes normally transmits environmental sound vibrations to the inner ear fluids.

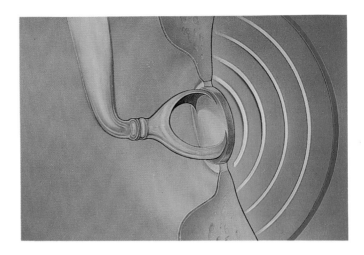

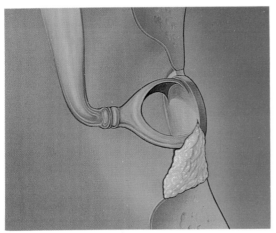

PLATE 7 Fixation of the stapes with otosclerosis results in hearing impairment.

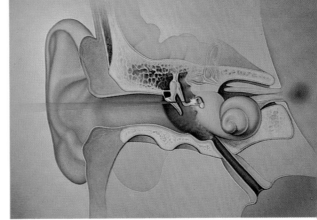

PLATE 8 The laser is beamed through the external ear canal onto the stapes.

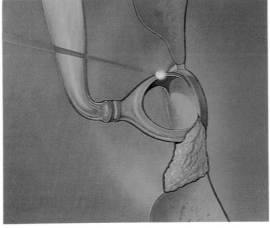

PLATE 9 Laser pulses are directed onto the back arch of the stapes.

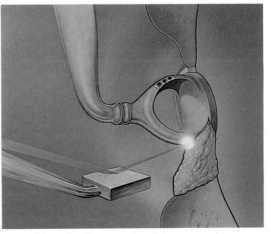

PLATE 10 The front arch of the stapes is vaporized by reflecting the beam off a miniature mirror.

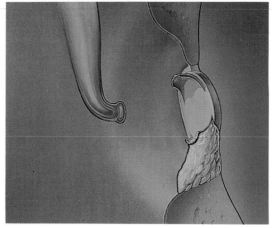

PLATE 11   The outer portion of the stapes is removed.

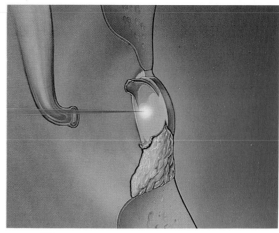

PLATE 12   The 250-μm beam is directed at the footplate.

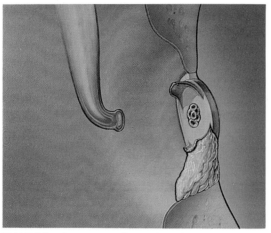

PLATE 13   A rosette of openings is vaporized in the stapes footplate.

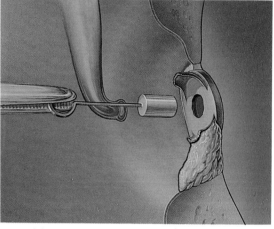

PLATE 14   A piston-shaped prosthesis is introduced.

PLATE 15   The vibratory pathway to the inner ear fluids is reestablished.

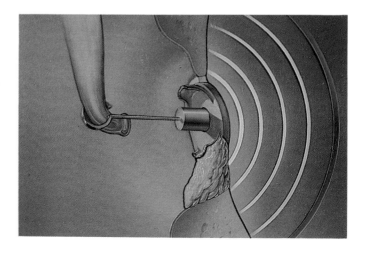

Medical illustrations for Plates 5 through 15 by Daniel Slotton, courtesy of Project HEAR.

delivered through transdermal probes that require minimal incisions of 1 cm or less. This is particularly true for those wavelengths transmissible through quartz fiber-optic waveguides.

Controlled tissue effects can also be delivered noninvasively. This is commonly done in the treatment of intraocular conditions and intradermal lesions by wavelengths characterized by high transmissiveness through the ocular and dermal media.

BIOLOGICAL EFFECTS

The laser is a very effective tool for the surgeon who understands its advantages and limitations. The surgeon's knowledge of laser science need not be as detailed as that of the physicist but should include a general understanding of principles of light transmission, reflection, scatter, and absorption. An understanding of the interaction of the various wavelengths in tissue components with widely differing coefficients of absorption provides the primary basis for safe and effective surgical application of this new technology.

The biological effect of lasers is a function of three elements: laser wavelength, energy density, and tissue absorption (Figure 2). For the surgeon, it is helpful to look upon wavelengths as the nature or character of the surgical instrument and upon energy density as the "dosage." The coefficient of absorption of the target tissue might be thought of as a sponge for this therapeutic light, but is more difficult to characterize and simplify.

Two important constituents of tissue absorption are pigment and water. In all but the most specialized of tissues there is generally a vascular supply rich in hemoglobin pigment. Other chromophore pigments, such as melanin in skin and myoglobin in muscle, are prevalent. All tissues contain water. Visible light from argon and KTP/532 lasers is well absorbed in hemoglobin, whereas infrared radiation from Nd:YAG lasers is poorly absorbed. In water, CO_2 laser radiation is almost totally absorbed, whereas the visible wavelengths and Nd:YAG laser radiation have little absorption. Thus, each of the surgical laser wavelengths has advantages and disadvantages depending upon the target tissue and the surgical effect desired.

It is not completely accurate to generalize about the relative amounts of penetration and scatter of these surgical lasers in tissue, because that is a function of wavelength and the specific absorption characteristics of individual tissues. However, if we consider a hypothetical nominal soft tissue with a mixture of tissue types found in the body, we can compare the general

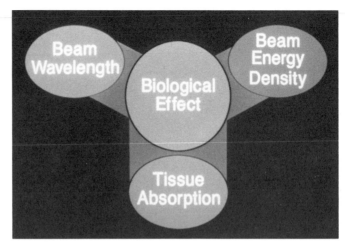

FIGURE 2   The biological effect of lasers is a function of three main factors.

scatter of these various wavelengths. In this hypothetical model, we would find CO_2 laser radiation absorbed on the surface with little forward scatter. The wavelengths of the Nd:YAG laser would have poor surface absorption and would scatter deeply into the tissue. The visible wavelengths would have forward scatter somewhat greater than the CO_2 laser wavelengths but significantly less than those of the Nd:YAG laser.

The thermal patterns in this conceptual model are also varied. The CO_2 laser produces a surface hot spot that creates a thermal front that conducts heat into the tissue. The thermal center produced by the Nd:YAG laser is actually beneath the surface of the target tissue, thus making it difficult for the surgeon to judge the ultimate surgical effect. The visible wavelengths have some of the surface heat effect of the CO_2 laser, especially once surface vaporization and some penetration into the tissue is initiated.

The CO_2 laser is an efficient vaporizer of tissue. The Nd:YAG laser does not characteristically vaporize tissue unless power densities are relatively high, but rather, it creates a coagulative necrosis within the tissue. The argon and KTP/532 lasers vaporize tissue effectively, especially after the process has been initiated. It is possible that as the target tissue begins to vaporize, a blanket of microscopic char particles is created on the surface and acts as a chromophore, catalyzing the surface absorption of the next quantum of visible laser light. The visible wavelength lasers are also good hemostatic coagulators. This quality probably derives from the slight scatter, which is absorbed in the hemoglobin within the capillaries and small vessels, thus creating intravascular coagulation. Carbon dioxide lasers have less hemostatic effect. This effect results primarily from the advancing thermal front, not because of any specific intravascular absorption of the wavelength. Whether the laser radiation is visible or invisible, the phenomenon that causes the surgical effect is the absorption of radiant energy and its conversion into heat in the target tissue.

The amount of heat generated determines the alteration of the tissue. At approximately 50°C–60°C, denaturation begins to occur in collagen and other proteins. At 65°C and above, denaturation proceeds to extensive physical changes, including coagulation. At 80°C–85°C, blood vessels shrink. This effect is probably due to the alteration of the collagen within their walls and is a component of the hemostatic effect of lasers. Just below 100°C small vacuoles are sometimes formed in the tissue as the slightly pressurized intra- and extracellular water begins to boil. Surface vaporization takes place at 100°C, and much of the particulate matter of the tissue leaves the surface with the emitting vapor. At several hundred degrees Celsius, the remaining organic materials revert to their basic carboniferous form and charring occurs.

SURGICAL EFFECTS

An understanding of these interactions between temperature and tissue is important to the surgeon in achieving three main surgical effects: coagulating, vaporizing, and cutting. In practice, the thermal boundaries between these effects are not as controllable as they are in a laboratory setting or theoretical contemplation, but the surgeon can achieve a predominant surgical effect by manipulating the one variable in the triad of the biological effect equation subject to change intraoperatively. Currently, lacking a variable-wavelength laser, the surgeon has a fixed frequency available and generally a fixed tissue coefficient of absorption as well. The only manipulable variable of the triad is energy density.

Coagulation for hemostasis is best effected by using a lower energy density, which is achieved by enlarging the spot size or lowering the absolute power or exposure duration. The surgeon can use this technique, particularly with the visible wavelength lasers and the Nd:YAG laser, for prophylactic hemocoagulation to prevent bleeding in small vessels and vascularized target tissue and to control small vessel hemorrhage if it occurs (Figure 3).

Vaporization is used to remove tissue mass primarily in tumor

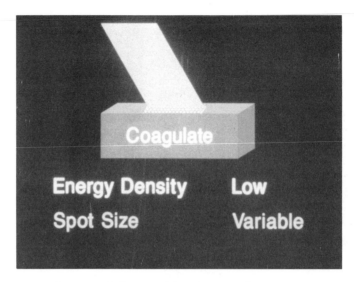

FIGURE 3   Coagulating to achieve hemostasis.

excision. The optimum beam conditions are a large spot size and high power density to achieve a higher rate of tissue removal (Figure 4). However, where precision is important because of vital adjacent structures, a high rate of removal may be undesirable for the preservation of those structures.

Cutting with the laser is basically a thin linear vaporization produced by combining a high power density with as small a

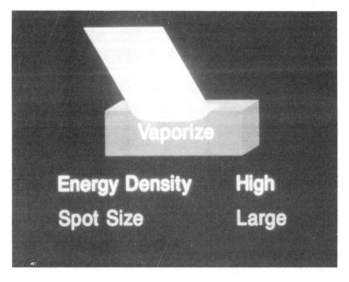

FIGURE 4   Vaporization for removal of a tissue mass.

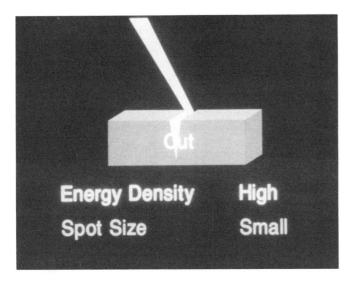

FIGURE 5   Cutting for incision.

spot size as possible. In a way, cutting with a laser is analogous to cutting with a scalpel, which produces a high pressure density. Efficient cutting is achieved by moving the beam at a rate that produces the desired cut, yet that minimizes secondary thermal effects in the adjacent tissue (Figure 5).

The surgeon has various instruments available for cutting and must select the one most appropriate to the task and the tissue. The only advantage to cutting with the lasers now in use is the degree of hemostasis that accompanies a laser cut and the ability to cut in areas difficult to reach with conventional instruments. Although the evidence is anecdotal, some surgeons report that patients say they have less postoperative pain when tissue is excised with the laser.

Safety and precision are maximized when pulses (for example, 100 ms) are used, since the damage caused by an off-target beam can be limited. The least safe use of a laser in surgery is the continuous beam, which, if it is off course, can significantly damage nontarget tissues before the surgeon can take corrective action. Between these extremes is the use of a train of pulses with a beam-free interval (for example, 100 ms on and 500 ms off). Such parameters allow the surgeon to view the effect of each pulse and aim the beam during the off interval or cancel the next pulse should problems arise.

Coagulating, cutting, and vaporizing are generic surgical effects achieved throughout a procedure by manipulating the beam parameters. When combined with an understanding of the anatomy of the area and the desired therapeutic surgical alteration, the surgeon has an effective new tool that can help enhance the quality and duration of life.

CLINICAL APPLICATIONS

Surgeons of all specialties can use lasers for coagulating, vaporizing, and cutting. However, in each medical specialty, there are certain lesions and conditions for which the laser is more commonly employed. The applications described below are not the only uses of lasers in these specialties, but they reflect the predominant current uses.

OPHTHALMOLOGY

Ophthalmology is the surgical specialty that is the most mature in using the laser as a therapeutic modality. In the late 1960s, pioneering ophthalmologists first applied the ruby and then the argon laser to prevent and control bleeding from retinal vessels. The visible wavelengths are well suited to this task, since they pass through the cornea, lens, and fluids of the interior of the eye with little absorption until they encounter the hemoglobin pigment within the retinal vessels or the pigment in a layer adjacent to these vessels. Here, the energy of the laser beam is absorbed, creating heat that coagulates the vessels.

Control of vascular elements in the retina through laser treatment has preserved vision in thousands of patients with proliferative diabetic retinopathy and senile macular degeneration. This latter condition is the most frequent cause of blindness in people over 65 years of age. The argon laser is also used to create "spot welds" to reattach or prevent the inner neurosensory portion of the retina from separating from the outer pigmented layer in retinal tears and the early stages of retinal detachment.

Glaucoma is a common condition that causes visual impairment. In this disorder, the normal outflow of fluids within the eye is decreased by malfunction of the filtering mechanism. The ensuing increase in pressure damages the optic nerve. The laser is used to treat these delicate filtering elements near the outer perimeter of the iris. Improvement in filtering with resultant reduction in intraocular pressure occurs in many cases, aiding in the control of this serious disorder.

In some patients, a visual problem persists after removal of cataracts because of opacities in the remaining lens suspension capsule. Short, high-peak power pulses (5–10 ns, about 1 mJ per pulse) from a specialized Nd:YAG laser are beamed into the opacified membrane. The beam creates a plasma that disrupts the membrane, thus clearing the visual pathway.

In experimental work now under way, lasers are being applied to refractive problems of the cornea. Excimer (gas) lasers are being used to make precise cuts in various patterns outside the visual axis of the cornea. As these cuts heal, the curvature of the cornea is altered and vision is affected. Another exciting and even more experimental concept is laser corneal sculpting. Using an excimer laser combined with a computer-controlled x,y,z plane delivery system, the refractive power of the cornea is modified by changing its outer curvature. The safety and efficacy of this concept are not proved. Two potentially serious impediments are possible mutagenic effects of the ultraviolet light and clear regeneration of the protective surface epithelium of the cornea.

The excimer cuts are not thermally derived, as is the case in other currently used surgical lasers. When examined histologically, the edges of an excimer cut show virtually no evidence of thermal damage. This "cold cutting" is thought to be due to disruption of molecular bonds. If shown to be successful, it would have other surgical applications.

DERMATOLOGY

The argon and CO_2 lasers have been used for years to treat various skin conditions. More recently, the KTP/532 laser has also been shown to be effective for these disorders.

The visible wavelengths work particularly well in the treatment of skin lesions that involve vascular abnormalities and in the removal of tattoos. The standard application is in congenital hemangiomas, which are purplish red discolorations of the skin referred to as "port wine" stains. They are basically abnormal aggregations of capillaries and small vessels in the dermis of the skin. Before the existence of the laser, little effective treatment existed for this condition. A lower power (1–2 W) argon or KTP/532 laser is beamed onto the lesion. These wavelengths pass through the relatively translucent epidermis of the skin and are absorbed in the hemoglobin inside the hemangioma network coagulating the vessel. Initially, the elimination of these vessels gives a pallorous appearance, but later, new vessels grow into the area and give it a more normal color.

The artificial skin pigments that result from tattooing are removed in a similar manner. Surgeons in many specialties use the CO_2 laser to vaporize and remove various raised skin lesions.

OTOLARYNGOLOGY: HEAD AND NECK SURGERY

The CO_2 laser has been used in the treatment of laryngeal lesions since the early 1970s. Although the throat is accessible with conventional instruments, it is difficult to work deep within the throat with long instruments. Lasers are used to vaporize vocal cord polyps and other benign lesions, but they are not generally used as a primary treatment approach for obviously malignant growths.

The KTP/532 laser has recently been used effectively in laryngeal lesions. Besides producing a very hemostatic vaporization, its smaller beam spot size is advantageous in making precise excisional cuts.

Like sight, hearing also has benefited from laser technology. The argon and KTP/532 lasers are used successfully in the treatment of the hearing impairment associated with otosclerosis of the stapes. The stapes, or "stirrup," is the smallest and innermost of the three bones, or ossicles, that transmit sound vibration from the eardrum to the fluids of the inner ear (Plates 5 and 6). Otosclerosis is a benign bony growth that sometimes develops adjacent to the stapes, causing its fixation (Plate 7). With local anesthesia, under a stereomicroscope, the eardrum is folded out of its normal position so that the laser can be beamed through the normal ear canal onto the stapes (Plates 8 and 9). The arches of the stapes are vaporized, and the outer portion of the stapes is removed (Plates 10 and 11). Using 100-ms pulses of 1–2 W and a spot size of about 250 μm, a rosette pattern of small holes is vaporized in the stapes footplate with an aggregate diameter of 0.6–0.8 mm (Plates 12 and 13). One end of a piston-shaped prosthesis is placed into the opening, contacting the inner ear fluids, and the other is attached to the adjacent ossicle, thus reestablishing the vibratory pathway (Plates 14 and 15).

This virtually vibrationless entry has several advantages over a manual technique: precision, reduced vibratory trauma to the exquisitely sensitive inner ear, and minimal morbidity, which is due to reduced vibratory stimulation of the nearby balance sensors. The procedure is routinely done on an outpatient basis, with concomitant savings.

GASTROENTEROLOGY

The hemostatic effect of the Nd:YAG and argon lasers has been used to control bleeding from gastric ulcers. However, this application is being superceded by a less expensive resistance heater probe employed in a similar manner through a fiber-optic gastroscope. The Nd:YAG laser is also used to necrose obstructive lesions of the esophagus in cancer palliation. Polyps and tumors of the colon in the lower gastrointestinal tract can also be treated with lasers.

NEUROSURGERY

In neurosurgery, the laser has been used primarily to vaporize solid tumors. The CO_2 infrared laser has been used predominantly, but visible wavelengths are used increasingly because of their superior hemostatic properties, precision, and ease of delivery.

Both visible and infrared wavelengths offer increased precision of removal, as well as reduced bleeding and traction on neural structures. These factors reduce patient morbidity and possibly also lower the incidence of certain potential complications. Argon and CO_2 lasers have been used to reduce intractable pain in some paraplegics by making precise destructive lesions in the area of the spinal cord that receives the roots of pain-sensitive nerve fibers.

GYNECOLOGY

At present, the field of medicine that is growing most rapidly in its application of the laser is gynecology. For many years the CO_2 laser has been used to vaporize areas of the uterine cervix that evidence a premalignant state. This laser procedure results in reduced bleeding and faster healing than other techniques.

More recently, minimally invasive intra-abdominal surgery has been possible by combining the laser with endoscopic instrumentation. The best example of this is the treatment of endometriosis, a condition in which tissue that normally lines the uterus is found ectopically in the lining of the interior of the pelvic abdominal cavity. At the time of monthly menses, this tissue swells and hemorrhages in a manner similar to that of the normally located endometrium of the uterus. Consequences of this condition include pain and infertility.

In laser treatment for endometriosis, a 1-cm incision is made in the abdominal wall, a tube-shaped viewing laparoscope is inserted, and the patches of endometriosis are identified. A 600-μm fiber-optic waveguide lying in a channel within the laparoscope is used to deliver the vaporizing beam to the target lesions.

This laser treatment of endometriosis is one of the best examples of minimally invasive surgery. Instead of requiring a standard wide abdominal incision, an effective treatment is accomplished with minimal effect on healthy tissue, virtually no blood loss, markedly reduced pain and discomfort, shorter hospitalization, earlier return to personal productivity, and lower cost.

GENERAL SURGERY

Laser applications in general surgery have not been developed to the same degree as in other specialties. Some general surgeons make skin incisions with the laser, but this is rarely done. Using vaporization in combination with more traditional techniques when removing large tumors is probably the most common use of lasers in general surgery.

This limited use probably derives from the nature of the lesions that the general surgeon encounters. These lesions are usually gross tumors or conditions that require anatomical reconstruction. Also, the surgical site is usually reasonably well accessed once entry through the incision is accomplished. Such problems do not lend themselves as well to minimally invasive and precision techniques—the areas in which lasers have the most advantage over standard surgical approaches.

PULMONOLOGY

Obstructive mass lesions of the lower airway in the trachea and the bronchial tree are treatable with laser surgery. Through a bronchoscope inserted through the mouth and throat, these lesions can be removed hemostatically, restoring the airway. This practice is used for benign growths and for palliative, but not primary, treatment of malignant neoplasms.

UROLOGY

Clinical application and investigational use of lasers in several urological conditions represent another outstanding example of minimally invasive surgery and the expanding impact of this technology. Bladder tumors that have not penetrated beyond the musculature of the bladder wall are treated with a minimally invasive technique through the natural urinary orifice. A viewing cystoscope is inserted through the urethral opening into the fluid-filled bladder, where the lesion is identified and removed. The Nd:YAG, argon, and KTP/532 lasers have been used successfully in this procedure.

All three wavelengths pass efficiently through the infused irrigating fluid. The Nd:YAG laser radiation penetrates and coagulates the lesion, which later sloughs off, and the radiation from argon and KTP/532 lasers vaporizes the mass. Higher energy densities are required for vaporization in this fluid milieu than in air because of heat transfer into the irrigant. Laser treatment of these lesions can be done under local anesthesia with the patient awake, whereas ablation with electrosurgical units is performed with the patient under general anesthesia because of attendant pain. This makes use of the laser particularly advantageous for the elderly, for whom other medical problems may make general anesthesia undesirable.

Urethral strictures that are soft tissue obstructions that impede the flow of urine from the bladder can be vaporized with an argon or KTP/532 laser wavelength. Small urethral stones have been broken up by a fiber-optically delivered short pulse (1 ms, 10–100 mJ) from a pulsed dye laser emitting in the green-yellow spectrum. This application is still being studied for safety and efficacy but is another potentially exciting and beneficial laser application in urology.

ORTHOPEDIC SURGERY

Lasers have been used clinically very little in orthopedic surgery. Orthopedic surgeons deal primarily with alterations of bone, cartilage, and ligaments. Currently used surgical lasers do not cut bone as well as other electrical and mechanical instruments. Although it is possible to cut bone with surgical lasers, they produce significant undesirable adjacent thermal destruction.

Investigators are now studying the technique of delivering lasers to the interior of the knee through an arthroscope that is inserted through a small puncture incision in the skin. This may prove a useful method for removing damaged cartilage.

CARDIOVASCULAR APPLICATIONS

The lure of using lasers in pursuit of the nation's number-one cause of death is strong, and many research efforts are under way in this area. Using an intravascular viewing catheter that holds a fiber-optic waveguide to approach and destroy an obstructive coronary artery lesion is an exciting concept—the stuff that dreams are made of. Whether this is feasible by using a laser remains to be seen. A technique to eliminate intravascular lesions will be developed, but whether it will be laser based, electrical, mechanical, or some other combination of techniques is not clear. Several problems confound this development. Obstructive lesions are neither simple nor uniform. They may consist of a fresh clot; soft, multicolored atheromata; a hard, calcified plaque; or a combination of these. The obstruction is irregular, and the restricted vessel lumen, if still present, is usually eccentric.

The highly varied color and consistency of soft atheromata and arteriosclerotic plaque make it harder to predict a consistent effect of a laser. Undesirable thermal damage to vessel walls may cause subsequent vessel constriction, aneurysm, or perforation. At the same time, adverse thermal effects on the myocardial electrical conduction system must be considered. Investigators are also studying the question of whether the solid by-products of ablation could block vessels. All of these problems pose potential difficulties.

Argon lasers are being used investigationally in attempts to vaporize obstructive lesions directly and to heat probe tips. Excimer lasers are being studied for use in plaque removal, but use of certain ultraviolet wavelengths is encumbered by delivery problems and the longer term mutagenic potential. Other wavelengths are undoubtedly undergoing evaluation for these purposes. Should these developments succeed, there will be a certain irony that a modality used first for its ability to close vessels should also be successful in opening them.

Additional experimental work is being done to treat certain arrhythmias by precision photoablation of areas of the conductive systems and to remove from heart valves any unwanted tissue that prevents them from closing adequately. The successful wedding of lasers with the recently developed intra-arterial catheter technology in cardiovascular applications could help considerably in mitigating the effects of one of our largest health care problems.

PHOTODYNAMIC THERAPY

The photoactivation of certain chemicals in vivo has potential in the treatment of cancer. A dye material called hematoporphyrin derivative (HPD) is being activated by exposure to low-energy laser radiation with beneficial effects on certain malignant neoplasms.

Given to the patient about 48 hours ahead of the anticipated laser exposure, the HPD becomes intimately associated with malignant cells. Upon photoactivation of the HPD, a photochemical reaction causes the death of the malignant cell hosting the HPD but does not kill adjacent normal cells.

Both 630- and 532-nm wavelengths are effective in activating HPD. The red 630-nm light penetrates farther into most tissues than the green 532-nm wavelength. However, 532-nm photoactivation may be useful in bladder tumors, where the lesions are superficial and usually multicentric and can be exposed to the photoactivator wavelength delivered by a fiber-optic waveguide with a diffusion tip.

The development of other photoactive entities specific to different cancers might add new possibilities for the treatment of malignancies.

THE FUTURE

At present, lasers have contributed significantly to the treatment of a wide variety of maladies. These applications and today's clinical lasers represent only the infancy of phototherapeutics. We will see other lasers evolve and take their places at the center of the clinical stage. Ultraviolet, diode, and free electron lasers all hold promise. Combinations of wavelengths, distributed both spatially and temporally, may provide tissue and surgical effects superior to those of single wavelengths. Miniaturization will enhance their usefulness.

Instrumentation derived from combinations of photoelectronics and other core technologies will produce still more alternatives to standard surgical approaches. Exotic and more highly specialized delivery devices will expand the surgeon's ability to achieve precision therapy with low morbidity.

Ultimately, these endeavors will advance minimally invasive surgery beyond our dreams. However, this achievement will be the product of human creativity and cooperation. The future of phototherapeutics will not be created by physicists, engineers, or surgeons alone but will become a reality only through the collective human resources of science, medicine, finance, and government working together with vision.

Lasers in Science

Arthur L. Schawlow

Lasers are nonequilibrium devices. Initially, scientists such as Albert Einstein and Albert Ladenburg, who understood the principle of stimulated emission, did not appreciate its possibilities—they were too accustomed to systems near equilibrium. In the 1950s it was understood that systems far from equilibrium could be produced. Since the demonstration of the laser in 1960, it has come to be used everywhere in science. Sometimes it is only an alignment tool, as it was in Burton Richter's 1976 Nobel Prize work, in which a laser was used to align the 2-mile-long linear accelerator. But often, the laser is more central. This paper describes several examples of such central applications of the laser, with an emphasis on spectroscopy—the author's field of specialization.

Ideal laser light is directional, powerful, monochromatic, and coherent. Some lasers approach these ideals more closely than others, and in any scientific use, it is important to pick the characteristics of significance for that application. For spectroscopy, which makes use of the absorption or emission of light when a material is irradiated by coherent light of the proper frequency, a key issue is the tunability of the light source. Thus, laser spectroscopy really began in the late 1960s with the development of tunable dye lasers by Schäfer et al. (1966) in Germany and Sorokin and Lankard (1966) in the United States. The organic dye molecules have broad emission bands, and tuning is done by introducing a rotatable diffraction grating, which acts as a tunable mirror, into the laser resonator.

This paper is adapted from a transcript of Dr. Schawlow's presentation at the National Academy of Engineering symposium "Twenty-Five Years of the Laser."

A fundamental difficulty in studying the interaction of atoms with radiation comes from the motion of the atoms. The emission or absorption lines are consequently broadened by the Doppler shift of atoms moving with a statistical distribution of velocities in different directions. Thus, much fine structure is lost in a straightforward measurement of the interactions. In the last 15 years several methods of overcoming this problem have been demonstrated. In one method, atoms interact with two light beams coming from opposite directions, and only stationary atoms interact with both beams at the same frequency. For example, a powerful saturating beam may be turned off and on, bleaching a path for a probe beam of opposite direction. The probe beam is thus modulated, but only when tuned to atoms that are standing still. Hänsch and associates (1972) at Stanford University used this method to observe theoretically predicted fine structure in the Balmer spectrum of hydrogen, including the first optical observation of the Lamb shift.

Two-photon interactions, using oppositely directed beams, were proposed by Chebotayev and associates in 1970 (Vasilenko et al., 1970) and realized by several groups in 1973. This method has been used at Stanford (Foot et al., 1985) to improve resolution of the 1S to 2S transition in hydrogen to one part in 10^9. Early laser measurements on the Balmer series gave only 1 part in 10^5, but were improved to 1 part in 10^7, at which point lifetime limits. The long lifetime of the 2S level would not limit until one reached 1 part in 10^{15} or so. This method has also been used in elegant experiments on positronium at Bell Laboratories (Chu and Mills, 1982).

In 1975, using a somewhat different technique, Hänsch and Schawlow (1975) proposed using light pressure to slow down the atoms. The radiation should be just below the resonance of the atom at rest, so that atoms moving toward the laser scatter the light and lose momentum in the process. The technique has been used successfully with sodium at the National Bureau of Standards and by Chu and coworkers at Bell Laboratories (Chu et al., 1985) to slow down a cloud of atoms, producing "optical molasses." Still other variations are producing quite surprising advances in precision measurement techniques.

In going from atoms to molecules, the spectra become enormously more complicated. With lasers, one can simplify the spectra by "labeling" a particular level. This can be done by pumping atoms out of or into a level or by orienting them. Then, when probes are brought in at two different frequencies, transitions are observed only from the labeled levels. For example, the complete spectra of diatomic sodium are quite complex, but with the labeling, one can see only two rotational levels for each vibrational level of the molecule.

Laser spectroscopy can be very sensitive since one can have repeated scatterings from an atom without destroying it. In my laboratory, as few as 10^5 sodium atoms/cm^3 were detected at room temperature, and as few as 100/cm^3 at $-30°C$ (Fairbank et al., 1975). The mean free path of sodium atoms in this case is greater than the distance from the earth to the moon. An experiment in Heidelberg trapped barium ions in a radio frequency trap, and by continued scattering of light off the atoms for several minutes, a single atom was observed (Neuhauser et al., 1980). By holding the laser beam on the material for a long time, one can do precision spectroscopy. Hurst, Payne, and associates at Oak Ridge National Laboratory have also developed methods for detecting single atoms and have shown a number of important applications to nuclear physics (Hurst et al., 1979). They have recently proposed a method for detecting the magnetic monopoles postulated by P. A. M. Dirac many years ago. The method makes use of a transition in helium from the ground state to a metastable state that should be excited by the monopole, if it exists (Hurst et al., 1985).

Very short light pulses produced by lasers have especially important applications in biology. For example, the visual pigment rhodopsin is known from Raman spectroscopy (also using lasers) to have a small part attached to a large part. The bond between them flips quickly from *cis* to *trans*, two forms of the organic molecule. The molecule is excited electronically and then probed with the short pulses fractions of a picosecond later. Cooperative work at Bell Laboratories and Cornell University (Downer et al., 1984) found that the relaxation time is about 0.7 ps, and that there are differences, depending upon whether the pigment is in water or heavy water.

At Lawrence Livermore National Laboratory, high-power lasers are focused onto small spheres of hydrogen to study the potential for fusion, which in principle could provide an almost endless source of energy. The scientific importance of such work is that it permits the study of matter at temperatures and pressures even greater than those at the center of the sun. The apparatus for this research is huge—larger than many accelerators—consisting of a master laser feeding an array of laser amplifiers.

In contrast to the short pulses, lasers can be used to observe phenomena that change very slowly. An example is the measurement of the motion of bacteria in a liquid such as water, where the Doppler shift is of the order of kilohertz. To observe this motion with conventional interferometers, using distance equivalents to time of about 30 cm/ns (1 ft/ns), distance differences of millions of feet would be needed. Photon correlation techniques are used instead, with velocities deduced from comparison of intensity correlations. In a typical measurement at 30°C, bacterial motion peaked at about 30 μm/s. Results such as this have helped in the understanding of how bacteria move. A different example of slow-motion measurement is the work at the Johns Hopkins University to measure the sliding and stretching motion of muscles. Again, this velocity is in the range of micrometers per second (Stock, 1976).

In geodesy, the relative motion of the earth's poles has been measured by satellite-ranging methods over a period of a year or so. Results agree with long-baseline radiometry to within a few centimeters and show a variation with time of about 600 ms of arc (about 20 m). The cause of this variation is somewhat controversial, but it is apparently not due to earthquakes, although perhaps to meteorological effects, such as air mass movements (Robertson et al., 1985).

Finally, lasers can be applied to a very puzzling experiment in basic science. In 1935, Einstein et al. (1935) raised questions about the completeness of quantum mechanics in describing reality. This has been expressed by the question, "Is the moon there when nobody looks at it?" Most of us are sure it is, but the question is not so simple on the quantum level. Following a theoretical analysis by J. S. Bell (1964), early experiments by Clauser and Shimony (1978) showed quantum theory correct, and recent experiments by Aspect and colleagues in France (Aspect, 1983) have been even more conclusive. In these latter experiments, calcium atoms were excited by photon transitions and then emitted blue photons and green photons. Detectors were placed far apart, and polarization was checked for the two. Since there is no change of angular momentum in this transition, the two photons should have the same polarization (or opposite if circularly polarized). Then, if a rotating polarizer is introduced, the variation with angle is different from classic and quantum predictions. The result appears to be too much correlation, as though there were a single probability wave rather than two separate photons. To make it worse, in an experiment proposed by David Bohm (Bohm and Aharanov, 1957), polarization was changed by the use of an acousto-optic modulator more rapidly than the time taken for light to go back and forth. The correlation still held. Quantum mechanics says there is no reality to things going back and forth; there is just one quantum system that includes the measuring devices, and the results are created by the measuring process. Of course, this is not transmission of a signal faster than light but only a correlation of probability, and many physicists say, "Naturally, it's just what quantum mechanics predicts." Others find it disturbing. A more detailed discussion of the issue is given by Mermin (1985).

These are a few examples of the wide range of laser applications in science. Many more could be mentioned. In fact, it is difficult to open any scientific journal today without finding a description of some use of lasers—if only for alignment. And it seems certain that still more applications will be developed in the future.

REFERENCES

Aspect, A. 1983. P. 103 in Atomic Physics 8, I. Lindgren, A. Rosen, and S. Svanberg, eds. New York: Plenum Press.

Bell, J. S. 1964. Physics 1:195.

Bohm, D., and Y. Aharanov. 1957. Phys. Rev. 108:1070.

Chu, S., and A. P. Mills, Jr. 1982. Phys. Rev. Lett. 48:1333.

Chu, S., L. Hollberg, J. E. Bjorkholm, A. Cable, and A. Ashkin. 1985. Phys. Rev. Lett. 55:48.

Clauser, J. F., and A. Shimony. 1978. Rep. Prog. Phys. 41:1881.

Downer, M. C., M. Islam, C. V. Shank, A. Harootunian, and A. Lewis. 1984. p. 500 in Ultrafast Phenomena, D. H. Auston and K. B. Eisenthal, eds. New York: Springer-Verlag.

Einstein, A., B. Podolsky, and N. Rosen. 1935. Phys. Rev. 47:777.

Fairbank, W. M., Jr., T. W. Hänsch, and A. L. Schawlow. 1975. J. Opt. Soc. Am. 65:199.

Foot, C. J., B. Couillaud, R. G. Beausoleil, and T. W. Hänsch. 1985. Phys. Rev. Lett. 54:1913.

Hänsch, T. W., and A. L. Schawlow. 1975. Opt. Commun. 13:68.

Hänsch, T. W., I. S. Shahin, and A. L. Schawlow. 1972. Nature 235:63.

Hurst, G. S., M. G. Payne, S. D. Kramer, and J. P. Young. 1979. Rev. Modern Phys. 51:767.

Hurst, G. S., H. W. Jones, J. O. Thomson, and R. Wunderlich. 1985. Phys. Rev. A32:1875.

Mermin, N. D. 1985. Phys. Today 38:4–38.

Neuhauser, W., M. Hohenstatt, P. E. Toschek, and H. G. Dehmelt. 1980. Phys. Rev. A22:1137.

Robertson, D. S., W. E. Carter, B. D. Tapley, B. E. Schutz, and R. J. Eanes. 1985. Science 229:1259.

Schäfer, E. P., W. Schmidt, and J. Volze. 1966. Appl. Phys. Lett. 9:306.

Sorokin, P. P., and J. R. Lankard. 1966. IBM J. Res. Dev. 10:162.

Stock, G. B. 1976. Biophys. J. 16:535.

Vasilenko, L. S., V. P. Chebotayev, and A. V. Shishaev. 1970. JETP Lett. 12:113.

Interactions Between the Science and Technology of Lasers

John R. Whinnery

In his history of lasers and masers, Mario Bertolotti (1983) asks the question in one chapter title, "Could the laser have been built more than 50 years ago?" The answer seems to be yes. Certainly, the principle of stimulated emission was known, and spectroscopists such as Ladenburg and Kramers understood that this could lead to "negative absorption." The technology of the 1930s was sufficient for some kinds of lasers—the relatively simple helium-neon laser, for example. But practical masers and lasers did not come until physicists such as Charles H. Townes, who understood the principle, were motivated to take advantage of the unique properties of these devices by their work with radar in World War II (Townes, 1984). Since that time, there has been continuing interaction between the science and its applications, so the laser is an ideal example with which to study the interrelations between engineering and science in a new technology.[1]

Nearly all new developments have a mix of science and engineering, but in some the science seems to come first; in others, the engineering. The science of thermodynamics is generally considered to have developed through the efforts of Carnot, Joule, and Rankine to improve the steam engine (Mumford, 1963, chapter 5; Bernal, 1970, chapter 2). In contrast, the major applications of electricity followed the scientific discoveries of Volta, Oersted, Faraday, and Maxwell (Bernal, 1970). The electrical example is an interesting one in its continuing inter-

---

[1]Although several historical examples are cited in this paper—primarily U.S.—there is not room for completeness and fairness. Readers seeking further detail are referred to Bertolotti (1983), Bromberg (1986), and Townes (1965).

actions over the nearly two centuries since Volta. Consider, for example, how the very practical effort to develop the incandescent lamp led, through the Edison effect, to J. J. Thomson's discovery of the electron. From this came not only the technological field of electronics but also the base for atomic physics and much of the science of the twentieth century.

A more recent example, parallel in many ways to the laser, is the transistor. Because of its base in solid-state physics, it is not surprising that the transistor was developed by physicists, who used the purified materials developed for microwave detectors during World War II. Later developments were carried on by scientists and engineers working together, with the result being both a new technology and also dramatic contributions to scientific instrumentation and computation.

THE MASER AS THE CRITICAL STEP

Although we know now that many lasers are simpler than most masers, the microwave amplifier using stimulated emission, or maser, was, in fact, the first device to use stimulated emission in a practical way. The science needed for this was, first of all, an understanding of the energy levels of molecules and solids, but the specific principle was that described in Einstein's 1916 work on stimulated emission. The technology needed was that developed during World War II for microwave radar—magnetron and klystron sources, semiconductor detectors, and waveguiding networks. But as Townes has described in his writings (Townes, 1965, 1984), his understanding of the noise problems of practical amplifiers provided the motivation for his seminal contributions to the field. Bromberg has described how other engineering knowledge motivated and became part of the field (Bromberg, 1986).

In 1951 Purcell and Pound demonstrated population inversion in a nuclear spin system by rapid reversal of the magnetic field.[2] Although a brilliant experiment, it was not intended as a practical device; the first practical stimulated emission device was the ammonia-beam maser of Gordon, Zeiger, and Townes described in 1954. This was quite a complicated device, so the three-level, solid-state maser proposed by Bloembergen and demonstrated by Scovil, Feher, and Seidel became the important quantum electronics device of the 1950s. The maser's promise

[2]Bibliographic information about work cited from this point on in this paper will be found in Bertolotti (1983), unless otherwise stated.

was as an oscillator of unusual stability and an amplifier with extremely low noise characteristics. Since the simpler parametric amplifier satisfies many of the low-noise requirements, the maser remains a somewhat specialized device today, but it was an important avenue to the laser.

LASERS—
THE FIRST ROUND

Beginning with the announcement of the ammonia-beam laser, there was speculation concerning the possibility of extending to the infrared, the visible, and the ultraviolet. (The names IRASER, LASER, and UVASER had brief currency for these respective ranges.) Knowing now the simplicity of some lasers, it is interesting to speculate about why it took so long to make the extension or, indeed, why the maser had to come first. One reason is psychological. In radio it had always been hard to make the extension to higher frequencies—from broadcast to ultra-high frequency (UHF), from UHF to microwaves, and from there into the millimeter-wave range. Consequently, most workers assumed the same would be true as one moved into the infrared and beyond. And of course, a good deal of understanding and technique had to be developed before devices that now seem "simple" really were so. Nevertheless, in 1958 Schawlow and Townes wrote the classic paper setting down the recipe for making a laser. The principles of that paper are still valid today.

It is also somewhat surprising that the first operating laser was a ruby laser, since it is by no means the easiest material to make lase. Ruby (chromium ions in an alumina lattice) is a system in which the lower laser level is the ground state, so that more than half the atoms must be pumped to higher levels before a population inversion is possible (or nearly so; there is some fine structure that helps a little). Nevertheless, Maiman's first ruby laser was not an accident. Maiman had worked with ruby as a material for masers, knew its energy levels well, and had calculated the optical pumping power necessary for the laser action. So for ruby, the laser was the natural progression from the maser.

Once the possibility of lasing action was established, other laser systems followed quickly. Many other ions in a variety of host solids were shown to lase. Lasers with neodymium ions in glass or yttrium-aluminum garnet (YAG) have proved among the most important. The first gas laser was the infrared helium-neon laser of Javan, Bennett, and Herriott in 1961. In 1962, four groups announced lasing action in the semiconductor gallium arsenide: Hall and colleagues at the General Electric Company; Nathan and colleagues at IBM; Quist and colleagues at the Lincoln Laboratories; and Holonyak and Bevacqua at the Syracuse laboratories of the General Electric Company. Thus, within 2 years after the first laser demonstration, three basic categories of laser—the ionic solid-state, gas, and semiconductor lasers—had been demonstrated.

LASERS—
THE SECOND ROUND

It is not surprising that most of the persons mentioned so far are physicists, since a sound knowledge of spectroscopy and either discharge phenomena or solid-state physics was required to understand the various classes of lasers. Engineering departments had become involved in the research on masers shortly after the announcement by Gordon, Zeiger, and Townes in 1955, however, and there was little difference between the courses taken by individual doctoral students in engineering departments and those in physics departments. Moreover, the major industrial research laboratories—Hughes, the Bell Laboratories, IBM, and others—made little distinction between the assignments of doctorates with engineering degrees and those with science degrees. So it is also not surprising that persons with engineering degrees contributed significantly to the next round of important laser discoveries.

Ion lasers remain the most important laser source for medium powers at visible wavelengths. Lasing transitions in ionized mercury had been reported in 1963, but in 1964 W. B. Bridges and colleagues at Hughes Research Laboratories reported many transitions in ionized noble gases, including the important visible and ultraviolet lines in ionized argon. At about the same time, C. Kumar N. Patel at the Bell Laboratories, in studying molecular lasers, predicted and demonstrated the high efficiency of the carbon dioxide laser with appropriate gases added. Physicists and chemists, of course, continued to make major contributions, as exemplified by the tunable dye laser demonstrated by Sorokin and colleagues and by Schaefer and colleagues, and the chemical laser suggested by Polanyi and demonstrated by Kasper and Pimentel.

Laser resonator theory is an example of a field developed by physicists, engineers, and mathematicians, often in collaboration. The open resonant systems proposed by Dicke and by Schawlow and Townes had been suggested by the Fabry-Perot interferometer familiar to spectroscopists. The first important analysis was a numerical analysis by Fox and Li, using Kirchhoff diffraction theory. Analytic solutions using the paraxial approximation were then supplied by Boyd and Gordon for rectangular coordinates, and by Goubau and Schwering for circular cylindrical coordinates. The latter analysis had been motivated by the problem of guiding microwaves, but it was also applicable to optical resonators and lens waveguides. Herwig Kogelnik then generalized this to show the propagation properties of Gaussian beams through a variety of elements by means of the ray matrices (Kogelnik, 1965). Thus, during this round, major contributions were made by individuals from different disciplines and often by teams of persons with various backgrounds working together.

DEVELOPMENTS AND NEW FRONTIERS

There was much development work to do before the newly discovered lasers could have practical use. Engineers, some co-opted from other fields and some graduated from the increasing number of quantum electronics programs in engineering colleges, naturally took part in this developmental phase. But physicists and others with science backgrounds did also. Bromberg, from her interviews with E. I. Gordon, explains how he first used his background in gaseous discharge phenomena to study the physics of gas and ion lasers in his work at the Bell Laboratories, but as time went on, he became increasingly concerned with development problems related to the devices needed for use with the lasers in practical systems—modulators, beam deflectors, acousto-optic switches, and the like (Bromberg, 1986). Similar shifts in interest occurred in other development groups.

The steady developments were punctuated by occasional "breakthroughs," again coming from contributors from all fields. The ultra-short optical pulse generation is one example. Pulse trains from the helium-neon laser were generated by Hargrove, Fork, and Pollak by the mode-locking technique, which was suggested in part by Lamb's analyses of nonlinear self-locking phenomena in gas lasers (Smith et al., 1974). Analyses of a variety of mode-locking techniques were made by Yariv and by Harris and colleagues. Shortly after, DeMaria and colleagues recognized that pulses as short as a picosecond were possible by passively mode locking neodymium lasers through the use of a saturable dye within the resonator. An important extension that produced trains of picosecond pulses from tunable dye lasers was demonstrated by Ippen, Shank, and Dienes, and was later extended into the femtosecond regime by a "colliding-pulse" ring configuration by Fork et al. (1983).[3] Still later, techniques of compressing these pulses by using the nonlinear effects in fibers were demonstrated by Grischkowsky and colleagues, leading to the very short pulses. Definitive analyses of the passive mode-locking techniques were made by Haus, Siegman and Kuizinga, and New.

Of the researchers abovementioned, Pollak, DeMaria, Ippen, Shank, Dienes, Yariv, Harris, Haus, Siegman, and Kuizinga had engineering degrees. A number of the key ideas in this field also paralleled ideas developed earlier for microwave radar. Although the parallels were sometimes not recognized until later, they nevertheless helped in the understanding or extension of the optical techniques. Thus, DeMaria noted the basic similarity of his passively mode-locked laser system and the microwave pulse generator demonstrated earlier by C. C. Cutler (1955). The pulse compression techniques, made possible by a frequency chirp introduced by the nonlinear fiber, were related to the pulse compression techniques of chirp radar.

The picosecond and femtosecond optical pulses have been applied to a variety of purposes, but by far the most important applications have been to the dynamic spectroscopy of fast processes. Because of this work, chemistry, biochemistry, and solid-state physics laboratories now have numerous setups for the generation and measurement of these very short pulses in order to study the extremely fast processes that may take place in organic and inorganic molecules and solids. Other examples exist, but this remains a textbook case of the way in which science can create a field of engineering, which in turn makes possible new science.

INTERACTION AMONG
THE SOCIETIES

The first article on the ammonia maser of Gordon, Zeiger, and Townes was published in *Physical Review*, but was later reproduced in the *Proceedings of the Institute of Radio Engineers* because of the maser's recognized potential as a low-noise amplifier or ultrastable oscillator. The *Physical Review* continued to accept maser papers for some time, until the editors decided that the field was well enough established that such papers should go to

---

[3]For later developments in the generation of short pulses, see the special issue on picosecond phenomena in *IEEE Journal of Quantum Electronics*, Vol. QE-19, 1983.

more applied journals. (The decision, unfortunately, came just in time for them to reject Maiman's paper describing the first laser.) There was then a shift in the physics journals to the *Journal of Applied Physics* and, after 1962, to *Applied Physics Letters*. The latter remains one of the most important journals for publication of new results from laser research.

The Optical Society of America (OSA) quickly recognized the impact that coherent light would have upon optical research and published basic papers on this subject in the *Journal of the Optical Society of America*. *Applied Optics* was established in 1962, and from its inception carried articles on lasers, optical resonators and guides, and electro-optics. Laser papers became an established part of the annual Optical Society meetings, and numerous topical meetings, such as those on ultra-short pulse phenomena and integrated optics, became the key meetings in those fields. *Optics Letters* was established in 1977 and became a leading medium for rapid publication in the field.

The Institute of Radio Engineers and its successor, the Institute of Electrical and Electronics Engineers (IEEE), encouraged maser and laser papers following its reprinting of the ammonia maser paper. These papers appeared either in the proceedings or in the transactions of one of the professional groups. There was, in fact, competition between different professional groups, as Bromberg has described (Bromberg, 1986), until the Quantum Electronics Council was established in 1965 with responsibility for the *Journal of Quantum Electronics*. The Council became a professional group in 1978 and a society of the IEEE in the same year; its name was changed to the Lasers and Electro-Optics Society in 1985.

Since each of these major societies established a firm position in research and development results on lasers and their applications, some vicious competition might have been expected. However, the societies cooperated from the beginning. The first Quantum Electronics Conference was sponsored by the Office of Naval Research, but later conferences were cosponsored by one or more societies, with the 1986 International Quantum Electronics Conference cosponsored by the American Physical Society, the IEEE, the Optical Society of America, and the European Physical Society. The annual Conference on Lasers and Electro-Optics is jointly sponsored by IEEE, the Optical Society, the European Physical Society, and the Japanese Quantum Electronics Joint Group. IEEE has also joined in the sponsorship of several of the topical meetings initiated by the Optical Society. Perhaps the most creative bit of cooperation was the establishment of the *Journal of Lightwave Technology* by IEEE and OSA jointly. This journal emphasizes optical communication systems, concepts, and devices.

There are other publications related to lasers in the United States, other societies, and other examples of cooperation. There are also parallels in other countries and international meetings. However, these examples establish the existence and the rewards of this excellent cooperation. Such cooperation between scientific and engineering societies is, of course, not unique to the laser field, but the degree to which it has happened there is at least unusual.

CONCLUSION

Two coupled systems can, with constant coupling, exchange activity from the first to the second and then back to the first in a time determined by the coupling, and so on, as is apparent in experiments with coupled pendulums. With diffused or random couplings, the energy that begins in one system may become more equally shared between the two after an initial transfer period. The kinds of couplings we have seen between science and engineering in the laser field have elements of the coupling example first described, but more of the second. Clearly, the richness and excitement of this field have come largely from the interaction between engineering and science concepts, between scientists and engineers, and between the professional societies. Progress in laser science and engineering is an admirable model for cooperation in other new technologies.

REFERENCES

Bernal, J. D. 1970. Science and Industry in the Nineteenth Century. Bloomington: Indiana University Press.

Bertolotti, M. 1983. Masers and Lasers—An Historical Approach. Bristol, England: Adam Hilger.

Bromberg, J. L. 1986. Engineering knowledge in the laser field. Technology and Culture 27(4):798–818.

Cutler, C. C. 1955. Proc. IRE 43:140–148.

Fork, R. L., B. I. Greene, and C. V. Shank. 1983. IEEE J. Quantum Electron. 19(4):500–506.

Kogelnik, H. 1965. Appl. Opt. 4:1562–1569.

Mumford, L. 1963. Technics and Civilization. New York: Harcourt Brace.

Smith, P. W., M. A. Duguay, and E. P. Ippen. 1974. Mode locking of lasers, in Progress in Quantum Electronics, Vol. 3, Part III. New York: Pergamon Press.

Townes, C. H. 1965. IEEE Spectrum 2:30–43.

Townes, C. H. 1984. IEEE J. Quantum Electron. QE-20:547–550.

Contributors

ANTHONY J. DeMARIA is assistant director of research for electronics and electro-optics technology at the United Technologies Research Center. Dr. DeMaria's research interests have included magnetics, acousto-optics, nonlinear optics, high-power carbon dioxide lasers, surface acoustic wave devices, picosecond laser pulses, laser radar, and chemical lasers. In addition to his industrial activities, Dr. DeMaria teaches engineering and physics at Rensselaer Polytechnic Institute (RPI) and other institutions. Dr. DeMaria received the B.S. and Ph.D. degrees in electrical engineering from the University of Connecticut and the M.S. degree in science from RPI. He is a member of the National Academy of Engineering.

C. KUMAR N. PATEL is executive director of the Research, Physics and Academic Affairs Division at AT&T Bell Laboratories. Dr. Patel's current research includes the measurements of Lamb shift in hydrogenic atoms, spectroscopy of highly transparent liquids and solids, and surgical and medical applications of carbon dioxide lasers. Dr. Patel is a member of both the National Academy of Engineering and the National Academy of Sciences. Dr. Patel received his B.E. degree in telecommunications from Poona University in India, and M.S. and Ph.D. degrees in electrical engineering from Stanford University.

RODNEY PERKINS, M.D. is a leader in the field of ear research and is a founder of Project Hear, a nonprofit medical institute for ear research and education. Dr. Perkins has a private practice in ear surgery at the California Ear Institute in

Palo Alto, California, and is a clinical associate professor of surgery at Stanford University's School of Medicine. Dr. Perkins received his M.D. degree from the Indiana University. Dr. Perkins is a founder and director of Collagen Corporation, a biomaterials company, and is a founder and chairman of Laserscope, a manufacturer of medical lasers. He is also a founder, chairman, and chief executive officer of RESOUND, a hearing health care company.

ARTHUR L. SCHAWLOW is the J. G. Jackson and C. J. Wood Professor of Physics at Stanford University. Dr. Schawlow's recent research has been in the use of lasers to study the basic properties of atoms, molecules, and solids. In 1981 he shared the Nobel Prize in Physics for his contribution to the development of laser spectroscopy. Dr. Schawlow received his Ph.D. degree from the University of Toronto. He is a member of the National Academy of Sciences.

ANTHONY E. SIEGMAN is Burton J. and Ann M. McMurtry Professor of Engineering at Stanford University. Professor Siegman's research interests include microwave electronics, parametric devices, lasers, and optics. Among his recent publications are *Microwave Solid State Masers, An Introduction to Lasers and Masers,* and *Lasers.* Dr. Siegman received his A.B. degree from Harvard, an M.S. degree in applied physics from the University of California, Los Angeles, and a Ph.D. degree in electrical engineering from Stanford University. He is a member of the National Academy of Engineering.

JOHN R. WHINNERY is a university professor in the department of electrical engineering and computer sciences at the University of California, Berkeley. Dr. Whinnery is a leading figure in several areas of laser research, including short-pulse optical phenomena. Over the years Professor Whinnery has also taken a leadership role in the training of students and the formulation of engineering education programs both at the University of California and the national level. He is a member of both the National Academy of Engineering and the National Academy of Sciences. Dr. Whinnery received his B.S. and Ph.D. degrees in electrical engineering from the University of California, Berkeley.

Glossary

*Bandwidth—The difference between the frequency limits of a band containing the useful frequency components of a signal.

*Coherent light—Radiant electromagnetic energy of the same, or almost the same, wavelength, and with definite phase relationships between different points in the field.

*Continuous wave laser—A laser in which the beam of coherent light is generated continuously, as required for communication and certain other applications.

Dispersion—In laser telecommunication, the spreading or broadening of light pulses as they pass through an optical fiber. Dispersion limits the rate at which light carrier pulses can be transmitted and decoded without error.

*Electro-optics—The study of the influence of an electric field on optical phenomena. See *optoelectronics*.

*Excimer laser—A laser containing a noble gas, such as helium or neon, which is based on a transition between an excited state in which a metastable bond exists between two gas atoms and a rapidly dissociating ground state.

*Gas laser—A laser in which the active medium is a discharge in a gas contained in a glass or quartz tube with a Brewster-angle window at each end; the gas can be excited by a high-frequency oscillator or direct-current flow between electrodes inside the tube; the function of the discharge is to pump the medium, to obtain population inversion.

---

*SOURCE: McGraw-Hill Dictionary of Scientific & Technical Terms, 3rd ed., 1984. New York: McGraw-Hill. Reprinted with permission.

*Hydrogen maser—A maser in which hydrogen gas is the basis for providing an output signal with a high degree of stability and spectral purity.

*Klystron—An evacuated electron-beam tube in which an initial velocity imparted to electrons in the beam results subsequently in density modulation of the beam; used as an amplifier or oscillator for microwave radiation.

Laser—A device that uses the maser principle of amplification of electromagnetic waves by stimulated emission of radiation and operates in the ultraviolet, optical, or infrared region of the spectrum. Derived from *l*ight *a*mplification by *s*timulated *e*mission of *r*adiation.

*Laser spectroscopy—A branch of spectroscopy in which a laser is used as an intense, monochromatic light source.

Maser—An acronym formed from *m*icrowave *a*mplification by *s*timulated *e*mission of *r*adiation.

Molecular beam epitaxy—A technique for growing single crystals of compound semiconductor thin films through the molecule-by-molecule deposition of material from a molecular beam. The structure of the film is determined by the crystal structure and orientation of the underlying substrate.

Neodymium-glass laser—A laser that produces intense light pulses in the near-infrared portion of the spectrum, specifically with a wavelength of about 1 μm.

*Optical fiber—A long, thin thread of fused silica, or other transparent material, used to transmit light. Also known as a light guide.

*Optoelectronics—The branch of electronics that deals with solid-state and other electronic devices for generating, modulating, transmitting, and sensing electromagnetic radiation in the ultraviolet, visible-light, and infrared portions of the spectrum.

*Quantum electronics—The branch of electronics associated with the various energy states of matter, motions within atoms or groups of atoms, and various phenomena in crystals. Practical applications include the atomic hydrogen maser and the cesium atomic-beam resonator.

*Ruby laser—An optically pumped solid-state laser using a ruby crystal (Al_2O_3) doped with chromium (Cr^{+3}) impurities. Laser emission occurs in the red part of the optical spectrum.

Semiconductor laser—A laser in which stimulated emission of coherent light occurs in a semiconductor when excited by carrier injection, electron-beam excitation, impact ionization, optical excitation, or other means. The most common form is the diode laser, in which electrons and holes are driven into a *pn* junction and combine there.